Releasing an Imprisoned Spirit

Removing the Seizure Focal Point

Karen Glumm

Hamilton Books
A member of
The Rowman & Littlefield Publishing Group
Lanham • Boulder • New York • Toronto • Plymouth, UK

Copyright © 2007 by
Hamilton Books
4501 Forbes Boulevard
Suite 200
Lanham, Maryland 20706
Hamilton Books Acquisitions Department (301) 459-3366

Eastover Road
Plymouth PL6 7PY
United Kingdom

Library of Congress Control Number: 2006934958
ISBN-13: 978-0-7618-3565-3 (paperback : alk. paper)
ISBN-10: 0-7618-3565-2 (paperback : alk. paper)

$\circledcirc^{TM}$ The paper used in this publication meets the minimum
requirements of American National Standard for Information
Sciences—Permanence of Paper for Printed Library Materials,
ANSI Z39.48—1984

Contents

Acknowledgements   v

Prologue   ix

Introduction   1

1 Noticing the Epileptic, 1991   4

2 Enter Historical Diagnosis: Flashback, 1978–1991   9

3 Imprisoned in the Mind, 1991–2001   18

4 Challenging the Spirit, 5/2001–9/2001   37

5 Facing the Skeletons in the Closet, Early Fall 2001   49

6 Releasing An Imprisoned Spirit, Fall 2001   61

7 Learning to Laugh, Mid-late Fall 2001   70

8 Epileptic Zoo, Late Fall 2001   85

Summary   101

Epilogue   103

Appendix One   Annual Seizure Report and Accomplishments   105

Appendix Two   Personal Seizure Description   107

Glossary   109

References   115

Acknowledgements

I wish to recognize a considerable group of people who helped me during the most difficult times of my life. My gratitude to neurologist Dr. Kevan Van-Landingham and neurosurgeon Dr. Michael Haglund for testing, recommendations, neurosurgery, and continued medical care. Thanks, for my "memory." Special acknowledgment to all my friends (too numerous to mention) for offering patience and support. I am in debt to all of you who were present and helpful these past years as I faced these obstacles with my health. It was a very difficult time and you all made it much easier.

My deepest respect to Ronnelle Paulsen, co-director of my dissertation. I remember the afternoon in your office where we constructed the human "hard drive"—our brain. You taught me how to delete the old "memory" files—my hard drive is not so overloaded. A note to my mentor, Gideon Sjoberg. It was through you that I learned the positive side-effects of being a "tortured optimist." I expect the "best" to happen in life. I believe it did—I'm still seizure-free.

Special recognition to Jackie and Ted Straub, Rosemary Hornak, Sam Carothers, Bill White, Beth Gill, Bill Tarlton, Pat Rowe, Holly VanRemmen, Lori Steele, Marchele Seaton, Susan Wessels, Ellen Graden, Ginny Knight, Gwen Clay, Nancy Borntrager, Jennifer Johnson, Jon Miller, Emily Gallagher, Sarah Russell, Jamie Lathan, Beth Mulvaney, Debra Horvitz, and Andrea Valletta for guidance these past few years and for reminding me that life does exist outside the field of Sociology. I thank you in particular Rosemary. I think you taught me how to laugh once again.

My deep thanks to Liz Wolfinger for introducing such perceptive questions. You are right, my insightful friend—through recovery I learned to accept my weaknesses, celebrate my strengths, and develop into a stronger and happier person.

On April 21, 2002 News and Observer reporter Mary Miller captured the moment. This article not only revealed my "secret" history, but served as the introduction to this book. Thanks Mary, for "waking-up" the writer deep in my soul.

I believe the greatest gift from my mother, Marge Glumm, was her notion that physical limitations were a minor inconvenience. Nearsighted did not stop me from "seeing" alternatives. Weakness with directions did not stop me from seeking a new life. Poor fine motor skills did not stop me from picking up the key to my future. I guess, thanks to my mother, I perceived my thirty to ninety "feelings" a month as a minor inconvenience. They would not stop me from my goals and aspirations.

A moment of appreciation for my father, Ray Glumm. Thanks, dad, for teaching me how to gamble. It was through you that I learned to never fold a winning hand in poker. Your spirit was with me as I decided to undergo brain surgery in August of 2001. I "called" even though I had a low card in the hole. I won the hand.

August of 2003 was an important month in my life—I celebrated two years without seizures and accepted the invitation from Ginger Wilson to join the prestigious faculty of the North Carolina School of Science and Math (NCSSM) in Durham, NC. Finally, the historical sociologist is experiencing the "great awakening."

As much as I enjoyed golfing I lost capability in the early 1990's. This loss had much to do with increased seizure intensity and side-effects of medications. Last summer I began to enjoy golfing once again. My thanks to Dot Doyle for inviting me to her Club. I don't think you noticed, Dot, but finally, the golfer teed off once again on your course.

Special thanks to Sue Stevens for opening her home to me the critical year post surgery. While at your place, Sue, I learned that every desert in life has an oasis.

Under the guidance of Marcee Toliver I learned the significance of Valentine's Day. On February 14, 2003 I, for the first time, celebrated love of myself.

A special hug to my intuitive friend Lyla McGuire. Indeed—I am redefining life. In the comfort of your home I learned to enjoy and cherish each moment of each day.

My deepest gratitude to Ellen Noonan for the treasured "Wizard of Oz" ornament. The Scarecrow grasping his "diploma" notes that I traveled the yellow brick road of life "brainless" for over forty years. You are right—I finally discovered my brain through my wizards: Dr. Kevan VanLandingham and Dr. Michael Haglund. However, that Scarecrow is not merely an ornament for my Christmas tree—it is my symbol of life.

A personal note to my sister. Thanks, Laura, for your presence and support during the first critical days of recovery. You might not realize it, but as you were helping me walk in the house I learned how to climb the mountain once again.

Finally, my deepest gratitude to Linda Tarkowski for noticing I was "drowning" in my epileptic condition. Thanks, Linda, for helping me build a bridge to survival.

Prologue

This book will attempt to describe my past epileptic experiences, current medical intervention and recovery, and future goals and aspirations. My main thesis is that the critical experiences of my past have had a major impact on my epileptic endurance, choice of neurosurgery, and recovery. Before beginning a description of these experiences it seems imperative to offer definitions of the four critical roles of my life.

EPILEPTIC

People with seizures face stigma in our society. People with epilepsy are incorrectly assumed to be far less intelligent than others or less able to hold jobs. People with epilepsy may encounter difficulties in obtaining insurance and driver's licenses, negative response of others to their seizures, inability to take medication as prescribed and changes in their interpersonal relationships. Having epilepsy may affect the development of confidence and self-esteem (Epilepsy Foundation of America 2002).

CHILD OF AN ALCOHOLIC (COA)

Definition

A child of an alcoholic is a child or an adult who grew up in an alcoholic family. Adult children are particularly at risk as they learned unhealthy coping behavior at an early age from the dysfunctional family systems in which they were raised. An adult child is someone who is grown up, capable, and responsible on the outside, but who is a frightened, hurt child on the inside. Adult children have matured physically and intellectually but not emotionally, because their emotional needs as children were not met in their painful families (Wegscheider-Cruse 1989).

Common Characteristics of a Child of an Alcoholic

Children growing up in an alcoholic household often fall into patterns of behavior that, as children, serve to manage the stresses and, as adults, keep the children locked in self-defeating behavior patterns. The following statements are characteristic of adults who have grown up in an alcoholic family. Although most people probably will identify with two or three of these statements, it is the children from severely dysfunctional families that identify with the majority of them (Wegscheider-Cruse 1989).

1. We guess at what normal is.
2. We have difficulty following projects through from beginning to end.
3. We lie when it would be just as easy to tell the truth.
4. We judge ourselves without mercy.
5. We have difficulty having fun.
6. We take ourselves very seriously.
7. We have difficulty with intimate relationships.
8. We overreact to changes over which we have no control.
9. We feel different from other people.
10. We constantly seek approval and affirmation.
11. We are either super responsible or super irresponsible.
12. We are extremely loyal even in the face of evidence that the loyalty is undeserved.
13. We look for immediate as opposed to deferred gratification.
14. We lock ourselves into a course of action without giving serious consideration to alternate behaviors or possible consequences.
15. We seek tension and crisis and then complain about the results.
16. We avoid conflict or aggravate it; rarely do we deal with it.
17. We fear rejection and abandonment, yet reject others.
18. We feel failure, but sabotage our success.
19. We fear criticism and judgement, yet we criticize and judge others.
20. We manage our time poorly and do not set priorities in a way that works best for us.

In order to change, children of alcoholics cannot use their history as an excuse for continuing behaviors. Past experiences have shaped our talents as well as our defects of character. It is our responsibility to discover these talents, to build our self-esteem, and to repair any damage done. We will allow ourselves to feel our feelings, to accept them, and to learn to express them appropriately. Then we can let go of the past.

Spirituality

Following Sharon Wegscheider-Cruse (1989), I believe it is the spirit that helps us think and feel and teaches us to love. Spirit is energy, spirit is love, spirit is conviction. The job of the spirit is the pursuit of truth: using our thoughts and feelings of love to discover truth and possess it. Our mind is built because of truth, and our heart is built to love it. Spirituality is a simple way of living. To live on a positive spiritual basis, people make four basic movements. The first is from fear to trust; the second, from self-pity to gratitude; the third, from resentment to acceptance; and the fourth, from dishonesty to honesty. By spiritual, I do not mean religious in any form or sense, but simply "goodness": the ability to love, to experience, and to respond, deepening our sensitivity to the world in which we live. Spirituality means the ability to find peace and happiness in an imperfect world. Acceptance, faith, forgiveness, peace, love and connectedness are the traits that define spirituality for me. Spirituality inspires a belief in a personally defined "higher power." My higher power is my future—a stronger, healthier, happier, and peaceful Karen Glumm.

Sociologist

Following Sociologist Charles Tilly (1981) I argue that a Sociologist conducts studies of society. Sociology grew out of the field of history at the end of the 19th century. As such, Sociology grasps characteristics of history but broadens the basic research question. The Sociologist wants to grasp a historical time period. When something happened will have a strong effect on how it happened.

Social Service Worker

A Social Service Worker enhances the lives of individuals with functional limitations and their families by initiating, implementing, and promoting quality services. These services include (but are not limited by) vocational, developmental training, and rehabilitation. Social service is an organized, planned assistance designed to promote social well-being assistance to sick, destitute, or unfortunate (www.ccarindustries.org).

Introduction

Serenity Prayer
God [higher power] grant me the serenity to accept the things I cannot change
Courage to change the things I can
And wisdom to know the difference

Reinhold Niebuhr

I am a child of an alcoholic who has experienced seizures for over twenty-five years. Two percent of adult Americans have a seizure at some point in their lives. Two-thirds of them never experience another. The remaining third—2.5 million people—have recurring seizures. They are diagnosed with epilepsy, a physical response to abnormal electrical discharges in the brain. Of that population, 150,000 to 250,000 are not helped much by medications, but could be cured by surgery. I fell into this crowd.

This book will detail, honestly, and often amusingly, erratic behaviors I have exhibited since adolescence and my gradual understanding and acceptance of this condition. As a child of an alcoholic, I refused to accept or reveal this secret with friends, attempted to cope with the condition, and eventually pursued treatment and correction. I experienced partial seizures for twenty-five years, but they were only medically diagnosed since 1991. I can describe a partial seizure including physical, mental, and social implications. This is fairly unique as most seizure patients do not remember the event. I have strong descriptions of mine. I also describe treatment and recovery.

Although I have experienced a few grand mal (generalized) seizures, the most common were "complex partial." While experiencing a partial seizure a person usually remains conscience but thinking is altered. My first grand mal seizure occurred when I was a baby and I experienced a few partial seizures

as a child. Patterned partials developed in the late seventies and occurred regularly at the age of twenty-two. Over time, seizures occurred frequently and
more intense. However, I never knew what these "feelings" were. Finally, after two grand mal seizures in 1991 I was medically diagnosed as an epileptic.
After several months of reading, I, for the first time, noted I had experienced
complex partial seizures (undiagnosed) since the late seventies.

For the past twenty-five years my mental "engine" has had only one gear:
reverse. During this time, I obtained my Bachelor's, Master's, and Doctor of
Philosophy Degrees. I have written and published three articles, have two articles in process, and I am writing a book (other than this one). During these
years I have worked for five Social Service Agencies, participated in the Illinois State Hospital Deinstitutionalization movement, drafted and received
several grants for social services, and wrote policy and procedural manuals.
For eight years I taught at a college in Raleigh, North Carolina. I taught nine
different classes, helped create the Master's of Health Administration Degree,
and was involved in six faculty committees. For the past three years I have
been teaching at the North Carolina School of Science and Math in Durham,
North Carolina. I have developed two new courses, sat on several committees, and worked with over 200 students to acquire College credits.

Walking backwards up a mountain sure was difficult, but I never let this
stop me from progress.

During 2000 and the first half of 2001, I experienced intensive neurological
testing to locate the seizure focal point and determine if removal was possible.
After brain surgery in August 2001 I now have two new gears. When tired my
brain in is "neutral." Eighty percent of the time my brain is in "drive."

As I have gone through life I have felt that time was my greatest enemy.
Sometimes I wished I could turn the clock backwards. At times I wished I
could turn the clock ahead. Many times I wished I could stop it. Now, all I ask
for is time, time to allow me to be the best I can be.

I invite you into this world—meet Karen Glumm the child of an alcoholic
who has experienced thirty to ninety partial seizures every month for twenty-
five years. My main thesis is that my twelve-step recovery as a child of an alcoholic (COA) taught me to cope with seizures, accept deficiencies, and pur-
sue treatment and correction. I knew the benefits of recovery and never let
dysfunction or physical limitations stop progress. I continued to seek epileptic treatment alternatives. On August 15, 2001 I captured the moment. I endured neurosurgery at Duke Hospital in Durham, NC. Dr. Michael Haglund
removed a tangerine size hunk of brain where the seizures were housed. During rehabilitation in late August, I felt my "hard" drive had crashed. However,
my hard drive merely "froze" and was "rebooted" in the fall of 2001, among
those I love.

I have been seizure-free since August 25, 2001. It is now time to relive the past twenty-five years. An experience is never isolated. Each builds upon the past and in turn affects the future. I always knew I was not meant to be a "member" of a crowd. I now realize this developed out of twenty-five years of "complex partials" and is celebrated by the testing of a neurologist and the scalpel of a neurosurgeon.

I can now identify this moment and place it into my personal history. It is time to once again climb the mountain: now in "drive." Walk with me.

Chapter One

Noticing the Epileptic
1991

FIRST DIAGNOSED GRAND MAL SEIZURE—6/22/91

Moving Day

June 21, 1991 (Friday) was a big day in my life. I was moving across town in Dallas, TX with a friend (Linda Tarkowski). We had found the type of condominium we searched for: two floors in an attractive neighborhood with a pool and hot tub. We had hired private movers to move our furniture and appliances. However, we decided to move most of our belongings ourselves. This was a hot day and I probably worked hard without rest or fluids. I remember feeling nauseous the entire day. I had difficulty concentrating. I kept telling Linda I was tired and did not feel well. I believe I was having many complex partial seizures this day. It was at this time I still called my seizures the "feelings." I was still in denial and thus I can not remember how many I experienced that day. After moving we went out for dinner—my favorite Italian Restaurant in Dallas. I remember not feeling hungry (despite all the hard work). I believe I was still experiencing complex partial seizures that evening. Thus, I was nauseous and did not want to eat much food. I drank a few beers during dinner. After dinner we went to our apartment to rest knowing the next day would be hard work as well. We didn't know what the work would be, however.

Emergency Room

Early Saturday morning (June 22, 1991) I woke up hearing voices. My bedroom was crowded. I couldn't understand language but I knew strangers were in my bedroom. I panicked. My roommate tried to calm me down. She seemed "concerned" but not afraid of the visitors. I could tell the men were

4

setting up a stretcher. This indicated they were paramedics. I figured I must be the patient since Linda seemed just fine. I was not able to move or understand language. Linda tried to tell me what was going on but I could only tell she seemed concerned. The paramedics put me into an ambulance. On the way to the hospital I was able to interpret Linda's message. I had a seizure. I was confused. Why would I have a first seizure at the age of 32? I knew this could indicate a serious medical condition: brain tumor or infections. In the emergency room the Doctor seemed over-worked and impatient. He asked me if I had alcohol earlier in the day. I said "yes I had beers with dinner." He indicated I must have had my first seizure because of the alcohol. I knew this was not likely. Seizures may be caused by acute alcohol withdrawal (i.e. alcoholism). I knew this was impossible since I had beers with dinner. He was not willing to listen and I didn't really care—I just wanted the appropriate tests. This would take place over the next few days.

Idiopathic

I was asked if I ever before experienced a Grand Mal seizure—of course I said no. I had not. After routine hospital testing (EEG, lumbar puncture, and CAT scan) my seizure was diagnosed as idiopathic—no known cause.

> I think today is the 23rd [of June, 1991]. I'm in Irving Hospital [Texas]—came in early Saturday morning—today is Sunday—at about 2:40 a.m. I had a seizure—woke Linda up—I woke up to Linda and two paramedics. Linda telling me it was ok and the paramedics to take me to ER. They checked me in for testing—to rule out the reasons [of the seizures]. I have been here for 40 hours—had a CT and then a spinal puncture. CT was normal. Spinal puncture is weird. On Dilantin now—hopefully temporary as they [physicians] rule stuff out. I haven't been in a hospital since I had my tonsils out [age 5]. I always said I wanted a non-serious convalescence—this is it—been reading, laying, relaxing. [Physicians] put me on seizure precautions. It is strange to have a [first] seizure at [age] 32. All tests were negative (personal journal).

I was discharged from the hospital after a few days. All tests negative—seizures probably would not continue. No prescriptions necessary. For awhile I believed this.

SECOND GRAND MAL SEIZURE—7/13/91

Until July 13, 1991. I woke up on the floor of my bathroom early in the morning. Linda was talking to me and once again I could not understand language. Finally, I realized Linda told me I had just experienced another Grand Mal seizure—now a pattern. We both looked at each other and said "damn." I was an epileptic. I was placed on a medication (Dilantin) and could not drive in the state of Texas for a year. My life was going to change—I was an epileptic.

> Saturday [July 13, 1991]—2:45 p.m. I had another seizure this morning—6:00 a.m. My life is going to change now—will have to be on meds awhile and I may lose my license—(I'll be fearful of driving even if I don't). I just can't believe this—seizures at 33—damn. It's hard to hope now—I'm seizure prone. Will see a neurologist but I doubt can give me the assurances I want—major adjustment time. I go back and forth—from being ok with this to being angry, sad, and afraid. I feel like a prisoner cuz can't come and go as please—I'm confused—how did this happen—how will I adjust my life? Damn I'm scared (personal journal).

DIAGNOSIS OF COMPLEX PARTIAL

I began to read more current medical research on epilepsy supplied by a friend. For the first time I noticed a new type of seizure: complex partial.

> July 29 [1991]. Been reading up on seizures—there is a thing called "partial seizures"—wonder if that could be the "feelings" all these years (personal journal).

Medical Description of Complex Partial

Complex partial seizures involve impairment or loss of consciousness. Loss or alteration of consciousness refers to a lack of understanding and memory of the event. An individual may be able to move about in a relatively normal manner, but is suddenly lacking in understanding. Subsequently, this person may have amnesia for the period. Many patients are partially receptive of directions from others. These seizures may last only a few seconds but most last for one to three minutes, sometimes longer. Individuals usually experience a period of confusion after the seizures lasting for a few minutes or several hours. This was called the "post ictil" stage (Leppik 2000).

Social Description of Partial

Over time I developed descriptions of my range of complex partial seizures. Before any seizure began (regardless of intensity) I would feel like I was on a plain and begin to rise quickly up a mountain. Eventually (one second up to thirty seconds) I would reach a peak. Once the peak was reached I knew the seizure would taper and recovery was next.

I learned how to describe "intensity" of the partials I experienced. I experienced three different intensities. A small/short seizure lasted five to fifteen seconds. I experienced little altered consciousness and no post ictil stage (thus immediate recovery). I might experience déjà vu, feel uncomfortable, and nervous. I was able to lecture, write, drive, think, and remember clearly this event and all activities.

A medium seizure lasted fifteen to thirty seconds. This intensity of seizure always had a post ictil stage lasting a few seconds up to ten minutes. I would experience a possible déjà vu and always experienced altered consciousness. It was possible for me to lecture and write during seizure and post ictil but many times I would struggle (difficulty with choice of words, remembering where I was and what I was doing). I would be very nervous, feel uncomfortable and fear. I would usually stop activity (when possible) and resume after post ictil. Memory may be altered. Many times I would not remember the entire seizure or what I was doing before the seizure began.

A bad seizure lasted thirty or more seconds. I would experience a post ictil status (recovery stage) of at least ten minutes up to 4 hours. My average post ictil was an hour. Déjà vu was possible. I could not communicate during this seizure. I experienced great difficulty speaking and understanding language. I always needed to stop any activity possible. I was nervous and experienced extreme fear with each "bad" partial seizure. I was quite uncomfortable during the seizure and post ictil stage. I would always experience altered memory. I would usually experience a lasting headache. Many times (according to others) I would "smack" my lips or try to "swallow" during seizure (swallow seizure?) I tended to grasp tightly what was in my hands.

Owning the Diagnosis

Sometime during the fall of 1991 I accepted the diagnosis: I was an epileptic. As strange as this may seem, the diagnosis answered life-long questions. Many friends and acquaintances (including medical support staff) were amazed that I was not frightened or angry because I was diagnosed "epileptic."

> This "feeling" guided my early adulthood. Whatever happens it will always be a part of me, of my personality—and a reminder of those who refused to understand: two doctors, mom, and friends. How can I blame them—it is my prison—how could they understand that (June 11, 1992)?

Most people did not realize I had been experiencing this strange "feeling" for over fifteen years. Finally, I knew those strange "feelings" really had a name: they were seizures. I always wondered what they were. I had tried to describe those physical experiences with friends and medical practrioners only to be stared at with implied disbelief. I accepted the diagnosis (to a certain extent), began taking medications, and followed medical protocol. During the academic year of 1991—1992 I revisited my past experiences with "feelings:" the years 1979—1991.

Chapter Two

Enter Historical Diagnosis: Flashback 1978–1991

REVISIONISM

It is time to revisit the past—rewrite the past. Historical research is conducted to uncover the unknown: to answer questions; to seek implications or relationships of events from the past and their connections with the present; to assess past activities and accomplishments of individuals; and to aid in our understanding of today's behavior because of past experiences (Berg 2001). So it is time to understand—to relive the first thirteen years of my seizure experiences: the "feelings."

CHILD OF AN ALCOHOLIC (COA)

Before describing my past seizure experiences I think it is important to describe some of my characteristics/experiences as a child of an alcoholic. In the Prologue of this book I tried to define and list the common characteristics of a child of an alcoholic (as defined by Sharon Wegscheider-Cruse 1989, 1981). Children of alcoholics (or dysfunctional families) learn to repress and deny their feelings. Negative or painful emotions are seen as "bad," and children of alcoholics tend to not learn healthy ways to deal with anger, hurt, or other emotions. The alcoholic family tends to have unwritten "rules." This was my childhood. A few key rules are important for my point. *Rule: the status quo must be maintained at all cost.* Thus, most alcoholic families are extremely rigid. *Rule: No one may discuss what is really going on in the family, either with one another or with outsiders.* Thus, the family has many secrets. *Rule: No one may say what he/she is really feeling.* This is a standard rule in

alcoholic families (Wegscheider-Cruse 1989, 1981). Thus, the rules of survival in an alcoholic family are: don't talk, don't trust, and don't feel. As
adults, we continue this pattern of denial. Adult children have learned not to
express—and often not even to feel—positive emotions as well as negative
ones. Joy, happiness, and pleasure are as thoroughly buried as anger and fear
(Wegscheider-Cruse 1989, 1981).

I acknowledged my past as a child of an alcoholic in the Fall of 1985 and
began recovery. I began work on the twelve step recovery program as a child
of an alcoholic (as noted in the Prologue of this book). However, I did not acknowledge I was an epileptic experiencing consistent seizures. Thus, I remained in denial of epilepsy. Don't talk, don't trust self or others, and don't
feel anything regarding "feelings" seemed to begin in 1979. I did not keep in-
depth notes of these episodes. Thus, I am trying (as best as possible) to relive
the first thirteen years of my seizure experiences.

NOTICING THE COMPLEX PARTIAL—"FEELING"

I believe the pattern of consistent complex partial seizures began in the late
1970's. While experiencing a partial seizure a person usually remains conscience but thinking is altered. I experienced a few partial seizures as a child.
The first partial I remember occurred during lunch in the third grade. While
in elementary school I walked home for lunch every day. While home one afternoon I suddenly felt sweaty and nauseous. My mother thought this could
be a cold or the flu and told me to stay home for the afternoon and go to bed.
Ten minutes later I was confused as to why I was home for the afternoon—
moments later I felt fine. I don't remember any other seizures—for awhile.
During the 1977–1978 school year I attended a community college close to
home and was working for a newspaper in my home town. One afternoon after work I went to a store in my hometown called "Clarks" (similar to K-Mart
or Walmart). While searching for college necessities (toothpaste, shampoo,
detergent, coffee filters, coffee pot) I suddenly felt nauseous and afraid. I was
hot and began to sweat. I left the store without buying any of the products and
drove home. I noted this experience as some type of "feeling."

> I had this horrible feeling. Don't understand this. Kept getting old ideas and
> couldn't really talk or understand others around me. I avoided people when this
> happened. What is it (Spring 1978 personal journal)?

I think this event was a clear beginning of my future as an epileptic. I just
didn't realize it that day.

"FEELING" INCREASES IN FREQUENCY/INTENSITY

Changes began during the 1979—1980 school year. I had several seizures this year and could no longer convince myself that the spring of 1978 "feeling" was an oddity.

> After classes I was lying on my bed studying and suddenly the "feeling" was back. I couldn't understand Darlene (roommate)—she was trying to talk to me. It makes me feel weird (Fall 1979 personal journal).

These "feelings" were frightening. Old memories flashed through my mind (i.e. déjà vu). I "sweated" (i.e. rise in blood pressure) and my pulse raced. My mind was "cloudy" and I felt fear. My mind seemed impaired: I may not be convinced where I was, what time of day it was, and what I should be doing. Many times I could not understand language. I didn't know what these patterns were.

> What the hell is this? I feel like an alien to this planet. I can't understand mom when she talks and she looks strange. I don't like the taste of food or smells. I'm tired all the time (Spring 1980 personal journal).

In the summer of 1980, these "feelings" increased in frequency and intensity. The physical side effects seemed to increase. For the first time in my life I began to experience fear of being alone. My family left for vacation in July of 1980 and I would have the house to myself. I was so excited about these two weeks. I did enjoy the time—for awhile. But the seizures continued. I think this led to new fears.

> I was in the camera room today and kept getting "feelings"—wonder what it means. I hate being in that room—I'm afraid there. I like the art department better—Judy [close friend] is there (Summer of 1980 personal journal).

I endured the two weeks my family was away—I didn't quite enjoy it as much as I thought—but I did survive. However, they came home one day early. They did not call me and notify me they were arriving home one day early. I woke up with lights on downstairs and heard voices. I was terrified. Eventually, I figured out it was my family. After this event I was afraid of being alone. As I look back, I think this began a new stage of my life. If a problem happened (break in, power outage, unexpected visitors) I may have trouble coping with the situation because of the "feelings." I didn't realize this was the reason but from then on (until post surgery) I was afraid to be totally alone.

LIFE WITH "FEELING"

I enjoyed life as a College student and social service worker. 1976—1991 was a happy time of my life. However, I now realize I experienced hundreds of complex partial seizures during this time period. I am quite proud that while seizing I was able to obtain BA, MA, and Ph.D. degrees and work in social service agencies.

I experienced complex partial seizures for over twenty years. During this time (as tough as all the years were) I believe three years were the toughest— years where seizures were most frequent and most severe. The first was 1980—1981. I started my MA degree this year while experiencing tough seizures. The second was 1990—1991. This was the year I took comprehensive final exams, began my doctoral dissertation, and worked as a social service worker. The third was 1998—1999. This was the year I was challenged by my Colleagues.

Obtaining Bachelor of Arts Degree with "Feeling"

I entered college in the fall of 1976 and graduated May of 1980. I believe I had several complex partial seizures as an undergraduate student in central Illinois. I can not document how often they occurred but I do have some unpleasant memories.

> I had so many "feelings" lately—like back to back all day long (Spring of 1980).

I continued to take classes, complete homework assignments, and enjoyed college life—seizure after seizure. I never understood the "feeling" but I did not let this stop me from experiencing life.

> Got up feeling sickly—didn't get up until 12:00 [noon]. Eventually I did my homework and met a friend for dinner at my pizza place (Spring of 1980 personal journal).

I did well as an undergraduate student. My GPA was 3.6 (out of 4) and I was going to graduate with honors. I was obtaining a BA in Sociology. This is not an easy degree to sell in the job market. My advisor (Ron Wohlstein) encouraged me to obtain a Master of Arts Degree. Eastern Illinois University (where I was obtaining my BA degree) offered a Master of Arts Degree in Sociology. I decided to apply for entry into that program. During the Fall of 1979 I took the Graduate Record Examination (GRE). This is a necessary exam for entrance into most Graduate programs. I remember having the "feeling" during this exam. I know I had to stop the exam and close my eyes several times waiting for the "feeling" to go away. I did well on that exam, applied as a graduate student at Eastern Illinois University, and applied as a Teaching Assistant (TA) to the Department of Sociology. I didn't know what that physical oddity was—but I was not going to let that stop me from entrance into an MA Program—with financial support.

Participating in Graduate School (Masters of Arts Degree) with "Feeling"

I entered the Graduate Program the fall of 1980. My plan was to take classes the first year. During the second year I would begin my thesis. During the Academic year 1980—1981, my complex partial (feelings) increased so much that I sought out medical intervention. I was going to break one of the rules: I was going to talk about "feelings" to an expert.

> Slept until 2:30 [p.m.]—can't believe it. Weird feeling back. Laid around all day.
>   I don't understand this—what the hell is going on? I have such old ideas (winter of 1980).
>   The "feeling" lasted so long. I was so tired after and felt weird for two days (spring of 1981).

Seizures increased—enter Medical Field

During the 1980—1981 academic year I saw three physicians—two in central Illinois and one near Chicago. I tried to describe the "feeling" I was experiencing at this time to a practitioner: "I'm getting this 'feeling.' I'll be doing fine and then I am confused and disoriented. I can't concentrate, think, talk with others, or work on assignments. Then it will pass and I'll be fine. It might last for a few seconds or up to twenty or so seconds. After awhile I can work again." As a result of this discussion, I received two inaccurate diagnoses and was "turfed." "Turf" is term used by medical practitioners when discussing cases. "Turf" means get rid of this patient: send this person somewhere else. This may be the essence of the delivery of medical care, the concept of the "revolving door" (Shem 1988). I remember hearing this term from physicians while working in a hospital as a Therapist in the late 1980's. I was turfed: inaccurately diagnosed and referred elsewhere.

Misdiagnoses

Two of the three physicians offered me anti-depression medication. I knew I was not depressed so I did not pick up the prescription or talk with them again. The third physician in the Chicago area offered me a different medication: Ritalin. I was a graduate student at the time (this helped) and I knew this medication was prescribed for attention deficit disorder (ADD). I was not given this as an official diagnosis but I was offered this prescription. I knew I was not ADD and never picked up the medication.

During 1981 the frequency and intensity of episodes increased dramatically. I once again explained these to a close friend—Lori Steele—studying to become a medical/surgical nurse. For the first time someone listened. I still remember her response: "Karen, that sounds like a type of seizure." I went to our local library to read on types of seizures. In the early 1980's the only types of seizures written about frequently were grand mal and petit mal. Anyone experiencing these seizures seemed to lose total consciousness and never quite remember the event. This did not describe my seizures. It was at this time I figured the "feelings" were just something strange about my body. Everybody is physically different—I happened to have these strange "feelings." I decided then to just cope with the experiences—cope but "don't talk."

I entered and completed an internship in the fall of 1981. I began working on my Master of Arts Thesis the spring of 1982. I planned on finishing the thesis within one year. However, I became so busy while working at Coles County Association for Retarded Citizens. I did not finish the thesis until 1986. As I look back, working and seizing full time was enough. I know I continued to experience the "feelings" but I didn't write about them in my journal for a very long time. I denied they were a serious condition.

Four Jobs in Mental Health with "Feeling"

From 1982—1991, I worked for four different social service agencies not knowing I was going to be a client in 1991.

In the spring of 1982 I took my first full-time job as a Social Service Worker. I was the Referral/Intake Coordinator for the Coles County Association for Retarded Citizens in Charleston, IL (CCAR). For the first time I started working full-time with the developmentally disabled. Most of our clients were mentally challenged—IQ measured below 80. Some of our clients had cerebral palsy, Down's syndrome, and epilepsy. I assessed client needs for placement in specific day treatment programs.

Our agency had a pretty strong library defining disabilities. During the first six months on this job I read all the material in our library describing seizures. Once again, none of the material described any seizure similar to my "feeling." The seizures described were grand or petit mal. Persons experiencing these seizures did not remember the seizure at all.

I met and served many clients experiencing grand mal seizures. I talked with client family members describing seizures and side-effects of medications. I witnessed many grand mal seizures. I felt sorrow for these clients—

not realizing I was experiencing complex partial seizures on a regular basis and would have my first grand mal seizure in 1991.

> It was a tough day today. I was home alone and kept having "feelings." Aliance (my dog) came by each time I had a "feeling" and laid her head in my lap and licked my left hand. I wanted to be alone (Spring 1985).

From 1985—1989 I worked as an addictions counselor for two social service agencies (Piatt County Mental Health and CareUnit) providing services for the chemically dependent. Alcoholics withdrawing from alcohol may experience a grand mal seizure. Most alcoholics are encouraged to take certain medications to prevent seizures when ceasing alcohol intake. Clients may still experience grand mal seizures and I witnessed many clients seizing during withdrawal. I was able to find medical attention and I felt sorrow for those clients experiencing unpleasant seizures. I didn't realize I was experiencing consistent complex partial seizures and would soon have my first grand mal.

From 1990—1993, I worked for Child and Family Services (CFS) as a therapist in Austin, TX. During the spring of 1991 I counseled a client experiencing "motor" seizures. These seizures seemed to last approximately twenty seconds. She would drop whatever was in her hands (groceries, glasses, baby). Thus she stopped holding her baby while standing. However, she would not take anticonvulsant medications and continued to drive. On a regular basis I coached her to seek medical intervention and eventually she did begin taking medications. I didn't realize I was moments away from beginning my own drug regimen.

Entering Ph.D. Program with "Feeling"

As much as I enjoyed working in social service agencies, I desired a Ph.D. degree in Sociology. I remember talking about this dream with a friend of mine (Ellen Noonan) in Champaign, IL many times. I moved to Texas in January 1988. I didn't know this at the time, but Ellen encouraged my close friend, Linda Tarkowski, to encourage me to apply for a Ph.D. degree in Texas. During 1988 I considered applying for the doctoral program in Austin, TX: one of the finest doctoral programs in the country for Sociology. I applied the beginning of 1989 and was accepted. I moved to Austin in August 1989. I was once again in graduate school.

My first two years went well. I was selected as a Teaching Assistant all four semesters. I enjoyed all classes and received mostly A's. It was a very busy time. I am sure I was experiencing many "feelings" but I have no notes in my journal describing these events. I was busy both years: full time student, Teaching Assistant, and part time counselor at a local social service agency.

During the fall of 1990 I took my first class with Dr. Gideon Sjoberg. This was a required theory class. During the spring of 1991 I took my next class with Dr. Sjoberg. This class was "Historical/Comparative Research Methods." This was my favorite class at the University of Texas. I spent extra time with Sjoberg discussing future research. Finally Sjoberg asked me to stay late one night after class. He asked if I had chosen a comprehensive exam Committee and dissertation director. Of course I said no. It was then he encouraged me to take comprehensive exams in his area (historical/comparative methods) and choose him as dissertation director. After an in-depth conversation we agreed I would take the comprehensive exam in October of 1991 and complete the proposal for my dissertation during the spring of 1992.

I finished my fourth semester in May 1991. The comprehensive examination was scheduled for October and I would study during the summer. I left Austin the second week of May experiencing "feelings." I would spend the summer in Dallas. I did not realize I would return to Austin in August 1991 an epileptic.

DRIVING WITH "FEELING"

On a fairly regular basis I experienced "feelings" while driving. I never fully enjoyed driving. I always preferred driving alone. If I had a seizure while driving no one else would notice. Therefore, whenever I was with another licensed driver I was a passenger not a driver. For many years my "feelings" were small enough that I did not have a car accident. However, I did have trouble following directions. Thus, I made many wrong turns. I was a much better driver on interstate highways. When traveling with friends I usually did the driving on the interstate and others drove in the cities. As I look back I realize I was having regular seizures while driving. I just didn't know what I was experiencing.

> While driving down to Nashville I had the "feeling" on highway 57. I was still in Illinois but suddenly I became nervous. I felt nauseous and I began to sweat. I was a bit confused but I was able to stay on the highway. What is this (summer 1986 personal journal)?

The seizures increased in frequency and intensity in the late 1980's. I spent an enormous amount of time on the highway without realizing I was an epileptic. During the academic year of 1990—1991, I drove from Austin to Dallas on a weekly basis. Without awareness, I experienced many complex partial seizures on the highway. I was still able to drive safely from Austin to Dallas. I didn't realize that I would voluntarily retire my driver's license soon.

"FEELING" DIAGNOSED AS EPILEPSY

As noted in Chapter One, I experienced my first Grand Mal (generalized) seizure on June 22, 1991. I experienced my second Grand Mal July 13, 1991. It was then time to own the diagnosis. I did not experience "feelings" for the past ten or so years: I was experiencing seizures. I had been afraid of the feelings but continued to deny that I was experiencing seizures. I had unwritten "rules" of survival: don't talk about "feelings," do not discuss what is really going on, and don't accept a disability. Thus, I lied to myself for ten years and now it was time to move on. A new life was beginning—I was an epileptic.

Chapter Three

Imprisoned in the Mind
1991–2001

Pyramids of Sacrifice:
The meaning of the pyramid to Aztec Indians was provided by its sacrificial platform. If the "gods" were not regularly fed with human blood the universe would fall apart. The Aztecs ravaged the region in quest of victims, recruiting them through conquest. Victims were lined up for the length of a mile waiting for their turn on the sacrificial platform. Still today, on the pyramid it is the "power wielders" who proclaim the myths and "peasants" who continue to carry the stones and pay the price in sweat and blood. Out of the power wielders come theories that propose the new calendars for human life—schedules for sacrificial offering.

Metaphorically, it is the "intellectuals" who define reality, develop theories, utilize power, and propose the new calendars for human suffering. It is the "followers" who are called in to suffer consequences.

Peter Berger (1976)

OWNING THE DIAGNOSIS

I left Austin in the middle of May of 1991 as Karen Glumm, the Sociologist. I re-entered Austin late August of 1991 as Karen Glumm, the epileptic studying sociology. Sometime during the fall of 1991 I began accepting the diagnosis. However, I continued a range of emotions trying to cope with ownership of this diagnosis. As I look back on this time period I followed a pattern called "stages of grief" outlined by Dr. Elisabeth Kubler-Ross [1969] (1999). She argues there are five stages of grief beginning with denial and ending with acceptance.

DABDA

DABDA is an acronym developed by Kubler-Ross [1969] (1999) to represent the stages of grief. "D" represents "denial" (no, not me, it cannot be true); "A" indicates "anger" (why me?); "B" suggests "bargaining" (yes, me but); "D notices" "depression" (yes, me); and "A" invites "acceptance" (I will endure). I did own the diagnosis but I did not accept the diagnosis until 2001. For ten years I continued to shift from denial to anger to bargaining to depression.

Denial

I followed appropriate medical protocol to treat my condition. However, I convinced myself that each seizure would be the last. This was denial. I never said I was an "epileptic." I did not tell most people I had seizures—only close friends. After experiencing my first and second grand mal seizures in the summer of 1991 a neurologist suggested that these seizures may be an aberration (i.e. they may "burn out" over time). For ten years I tried to convince myself that this was true. I may have seizures for awhile but eventually I told myself I would be "cured." I was in denial.

Anger

I did experience anger a few times. I think my mother was angry at herself thinking the high fever I experienced as a baby inspired seizures. However, I was never angry at my mother but I was angry at the brain. I took medications, visited physicians and neurologists, slept more than average, and reduced alcohol intake. Why were the seizures getting worse even when I added new medications? I did stuff anger away though—I didn't stay angry very often or very long. I think bargaining was the most frequent stage. In fact, I think a connection between anger and bargaining helped my "drive." I wouldn't let my brain stop accomplishments and continued to "bargain" with my soul to continue achieving while experiencing so many seizures every month.

Bargaining

On a fairly regular basis I "bargained." Each morning after waking up I would tell myself "ok, I have seizures, but I could make myself better." I believed if I slept well and took medications on a regular basis the seizures would "go away." I tried this pattern for ten years. I increased medications and sleep patterns on a regular basis. I checked into Duke Hospital in 2001 to "bargain." I would follow the directions, receive testing, and accept new medications.

Then the seizures would decrease. I still did not "own" the diagnosis and contemplate surgery until late July 2001.

Depression

I did not realize at the time but I was depressed on a periodic basis. I think this started about 1998. I stopped driving because a severe complex partial seizure resulted in a car accident (I drove my car off the road into a tree). Medications were increased but seizures did not decrease in intensity or frequency. I began having trouble at work. Co-workers seemed to be embarrassed working with someone experiencing seizures. My life was very trying at this time and I started sleeping more every day to avoid "reality."

Acceptance

To a certain extent I did accept my diagnosis. I did take medications on a regular basis, reduced alcohol intake, slept well, and saw physicians on a regular basis. However, I never fully accepted myself as an "epileptic." Not entirely—but I did try.

Borrowed COA 12 Step Recovery Program

I searched for "mental" survival during the fall of 1991. I was diagnosed an "epileptic." I was deep in graduate studies at the University of Texas. I was preparing for comprehensive exams and beginning my dissertation. I didn't have time for a severe disability. I wanted to endure—diagnosis or not. I borrowed my COA 12 step recovery program to accept epilepsy. I believe this program helped me accomplish a great deal. I never gave up hope—I coped with seizures, worked as a therapist, and obtained my Ph.D.

> The First Step of Recovery for Adult Children of Alcoholics
> (www.geocities.com/howitworks2001/)
> We acknowledge and accept that we are powerless in controlling the lives of others, and that trying to control others makes our lives unmanageable.

I attempted to take the first step. I could not (at this time) totally admit I was powerless over my seizures. I tried to "fight back" as much as possible. I am a "tortured optimist"—I always believe the "best" will happen in any situation.

Tortured Optimist

Positive view about humanity's prospects. Sociology can help attain a more humane world. "Tortured" arrives with respect to the present: the optimistic conception of justice and fairness with respect to the way in which organizational power is wielded fails. Brutality of human conditions continue (Sjoberg 1989).

Coping with Seizures

My life changed when I was diagnosed as an epileptic. I could no longer drive in the state of Texas (for at least one year), regularly took an anti-seizure medication (Tegretol) and frequently visited physicians for medication blood levels. However, from 1991—2001, I continued to seize on a fairly regular basis. Seizures were not controlled by medication. I did not complain, however. I attempted to cope with continuing seizures. I figured the seizures could be worse without the medication. I took medications as directed, saw my physician on a regular basis, and consistently had my blood tested (to maintain medication blood levels). I would not allow the seizures to stop my progress in my doctoral program. I started recording each seizure I experienced. I always thought each one could be the "last."

> I have had fewer seizures recently—what a rush. Haven't had a partial at all since 5/26 and not a bad one since 5/15—the "feeling" guided my early adulthood—now—who knows—could become part of my past (June 11, 1992).

Until surgery, however, that never happened. Each year, according to my records, I experienced between 200 and 400 seizures. I recorded the length and intensity of each seizure I experienced. (Please see appendix one for a record of these seizures). As I look back on these ten years I realize that seizures were more frightening than "feelings." I was diagnosed as an epileptic: I could not lie to myself any longer. I once believed that the "feelings" were just a part of my body—nothing real serious. I never recorded "feelings" and thus I was convinced they were infrequent. However, beginning 1991 I had a medical diagnosis and this was serious. I was an epileptic. I recorded each seizure and thus episodes were more frequent than "feelings." I began recording each episode in my journal on August 6, 1991. On March 14, 1993 I realized episodes were so frequent they needed to be recorded in a notebook (a notebook that included a list of upcoming events). On December 13, 1994 (because of frequency) I needed a notebook that only recorded episodes. Denial was beginning to fade. My life focused on seizures. If I didn't write in the notebook it was a good day.

Side effects of Medications

All seizure medications have possible side effects. For some patients side effects are minimal. For others side effects are severe. I believe I experienced

the severe side effects of many medications. My first medication was Tegretol. At this time period (early 1990's) Tegretol was considered the ideal medication for those experiencing partial seizures: my main seizure condition.
The main side effect of Tegretol was double vision. On a daily basis (usually
in the morning or when dehydrated) I experienced double vision. I never
complained of this experience. I figured double vision was not as bad as more
severe seizures. However, I continued to seize on a regular basis (to my
knowledge about twenty or more per month) and I experienced double vision
every day. Crossing streets, using stairwells, reading, and writing were difficult while experiencing double vision. Many patients may have complained
more than I did and I would encourage current patients to voice discomfort.
However, child of an alcoholic that I was, I endured double vision on a consistent basis until the medication was removed in 2001 under advisement of
Dr. Kevan VanLandingham.

Because I continued to seize while on Tegretol I was encouraged in 1998
to add-on another medication: Depakote. The primary side effect of this medication was nausea. I took this medication for several years (1998–2001). For
the first several months the nausea was the worst. I spent every evening on
the floor of my bathroom throwing up. I was dizzy, nauseous, and sick. One
friend encouraged me to smoke marijuana if I was so sick I could not stand
up. Apparently, the nausea was not a result of an upset stomach—my brain
was uncomfortable as a result of depakote and seizures. Therefore, marijuana
would help relax the brain. I needed to smoke marijuana several times during
the first six months of the medication. Over time I somewhat adjusted to Depakote. However, nausea never was totally controlled. For the first time in my
life eating was a chore. I learned to count calories every day to ensure I ate
enough food. I had difficulty eating strong foods. I no longer was attracted to
my favorite Italian foods. I couldn't stand the smell of garlic, olive oil, or any
fried foods. A friend of mine encouraged me to drink ginger ale to quite nausea. She was right. I needed to eat every day so many times drank ginger ale
to calm nausea. While visiting a friend, Lyla McGuire, in Illinois in 2000 I
was so nauseas late one night I was unable to sleep. I tried drinking water but
this did not help. Nausea increased. Finally, Lyla's husband Tony heard me
pacing and ask what I needed. I stated that the only "drug" that could help
was ginger ale. Tony (after 1:00 a.m.) searched his hometown until he found
me ginger ale. This beverage helped me quiet the nausea and I was able to fall
asleep an hour later. This was my pattern (every other week or so) for over
three years. This medication regimen was very difficult but necessary. Because of lack of understanding of epilepsy, because of denial of condition, because of side-effects of medications, many epileptics are not medication com-

pliant. I was. As unpleasant as the medications were, increased seizure behavior (grand mal or more frequent partials) was worse. I had insight.

Insight

Insight is a self-understanding as to the motives and reasons behind one's action or one's condition (On-line Dictionary:cancerweb.ncl.ac.uk/cgi-bin/omd 1997–2002). I accepted my diagnosis of epilepsy. This was the first step into recovery. My twelve step children of alcoholic recovery program helped me own my diagnosis.

I retired my driver's license, continued on prescription regimen, tolerated side-effects of medications, and continued to seize on a regular basis. I knew it could be worse without treatment (continued medications, monitor results, test for alternatives). I learned (as much as possible) to live with seizures and construct a lifestyle.

If I felt an "aura" or a seizure began I tried (if possible) to reduce activity. Before mental confusion increased I tried to stop running water, turn off the stove, stop eating or drinking, and try to sit down. I would try to leave stairwells, leave classrooms, end a phone call, and seek a safe place. My safest place was at home. The next safest was in my office on campus. Next on the list was alone in rooms (so I would not have to verbally communicate). Many times the seizure escalated so quickly that I did not have time to stop activities or seek a safe place. Hence I did have a car accident, dropped many objects, spilled drinks on myself or the floor, and fell a few times.

During the mid to late 1990's my memory was weakening as seizures increased in intensity. I had insight: I knew this was happening and I (on a continuous basis) fought cranial degeneration as a result of seizure intensity. I created "mind games" to exercise my brain daily. On a regular basis (as I woke up, in the shower, while eating, while exercising, before falling to sleep) I asked my favorite movies and actors, special dates, or names of friends or favorites foods. I would pull up memories on all vacations, cities I visited, and reviewed the details of old friendships. I continued to visit museums and watch TV shows on history and nature. I continue to work my brain. I continued to read, write, think, lecture, and travel. I continued to teach statistics and research methods. I continued to keep a journal to record all activities and experiences.

As I look back on this time period I kept my brain "in shape." I had insight. I was losing some memory but never stopped fighting. Thus, my capabilities remained quite high. I didn't realize this at the time, but this was excellent cranial physical therapy.

RITUALISTIC BEHAVIOR 1991–2001

As I review the years 1991 to 2001 (official medical diagnosis until removal of focal point) I can see a pattern of ritual behavior. I believe I was somewhat aware of this pattern but I did not know how to reduce my ritualistic behavior. I now realize that I never knew when or where I would have seizures. I just knew they were frequent, frightening, and challenging. Thus, I had patterns of predictable behavior/chores so I knew what and when I would perform necessary tasks. What is strange is that I had been experiencing seizures on a somewhat frequent basis since the late 1970's. However, I did not know they were seizures—they were "feelings" and thus did not force me into ritualistic behavior. Seizures did.

> I seem out of balance now—I don't like the way my day flows—I feel too much isolation. I don't seem to feel much happiness—I feel much more sensitive than before I knew of the seizures. One of the things that I learned with the Ph.D. is that I will be successful—a project will be completed if I just continue—small steps at a time (September 10, 1995).

Planning Schedule/Recording Accomplishments

On a regular basis I planned my daily schedule well in advance. I also recorded every accomplishment. I am aware that most people are busy (as a result of multiple roles such as parent, employee, friend, and partner) and thus plan schedules on a regular basis. However, sometime in late 1991 (after I was officially diagnosed an epileptic) I began planning my daily schedule in-depth. Every night I wrote down what I had done and what should be accomplished the next day. It was during this year I began doubting my "memory." Thus, after seizing I could review the schedule to see what I had done and what should be done next. I never gave myself a "day off" unless I had a very severe partial seizure. This type of seizure would zap most of my mental strength for the entire day and leave a severe headache. These were the only days I gave myself a vacation.

Projects Completed Early

Throughout my adult life I have completed projects early. I have never tested deadlines constructed by others (government, jobs, friends). I have turned in required material early for over twenty-five years. Because I experienced up to sixty seizures per month, because I never knew when they would occur, and because I could never anticipate the severity I never tested deadlines. If I waited until the last moment to turn in a project and I then experienced a seizure the project may be delinquent. If this occurred more than once, it could call into question my professional capabilities.

This ambition spread throughout my life. As a student I read books, studied for exams, and finished papers and projects well before the due date. I arrived at airports to board a plane or pick up travelers well before departure or arrival times. I arrived in class early as a student or faculty member. I graded exams and turned in grades early. I woke up early each morning, showered, dressed, and ate well before I would need to leave. I arrived early everywhere for twenty-five years. I arrived at all scheduled meetings early. I ordered books early for every class I ever taught. I wrote tests early for every class I taught and turned them into the copy center before most other faculty members.

I never followed deadlines imposed by others: I wrote my own deadlines. My deadlines were constructed on a seizure-oriented clock. Thus, for most of my life I was early. My motto seemed to be: hurry up to wait. This seemed to be better than pressing imposed deadlines. If I followed other's deadlines I may have been late with projects as a result of consistent seizures.

Calories/Meals

In 1998 I added a new ritual: counting calories regularly. A new medication was added to my drug regimen this year: Depakote. Depakote challenges appetite for most of those consuming the drug. I was on this drug for four years and was consistently nauseous. I did not have an appetite—I was never hungry. I knew I had to consume as many calories as possible to reduce nausea. I also knew I needed to consume fat and protein calories. For whatever reason, these were the toughest calories to consume but were necessary to breakdown my medications. Every day I recorded in a notebook how many and what type of calories I consumed. I still have that notebook. I still have the notebook that documented each seizure. These are part of my epileptic history.

Fluids

In late 1991 I was prescribed Tegretol. I stayed on Tegretol for ten years. The most common side-effect was double vision. This tended to happen mid morning and mid afternoon. This was about the time I hit the "peak" time of my morning and afternoon doses. Consumption of fluids (especially water) can reduce the double vision side effect. On a regular basis I consumed as much water as possible. So much so that I carried at least two bottles of water everywhere I went. I was one of the fewest passengers on airplanes, buses, and taxis carrying a few bottles of water. Friends were amused that I would be headed off to a restaurant carrying a water bottle. However, as much as I tried, I could never totally control the double vision side effect of Tegretol. As I look back on this time period, I endured the side effects too long. The medication did not offer enough support to endure side effects. This was one of the first drugs Dr. VanLandingham encouraged me to discontinue.

Sleep

In late 1991 I began pressing additional sleep. I was learning much about seizure lifestyles. I knew that "exhausted" brains were more likely to seize. In fact, a healthy brain may seize if awake a few days in a row. An epileptic has a low seizure threshold and thus is a likely candidate for a seizure with a tired brain. As much as possible I tried to sleep nine hours every night. I tried to take a nap many afternoons every week. I convinced myself that my seizures would taper if I slept as much as possible. I think I slept a good deal of my life away from 1991–2001. Maybe I did help my brain but I did continue to experience at least thirty seizures a month—even with ten or eleven hours of sleep most days.

ACCOMPLISHMENTS

My diagnosis did not stop me from my goals and aspirations. I never even considered dropping out of my doctoral program or quitting my job as a therapist. I continued my pattern. I didn't see any difference. I knew I no longer had "feelings"—I had seizures. For over twenty years seizures were a part of my life. If friends or cohorts knew I was seizing they would tell me how sorry they were that I was having so many seizures. I believe people expressed sorrow because they thought seizures were tragic. For me, seizures were a fact of life.

Student/Teaching Assistant

I arrived on campus at the University of Texas in late August. I was a full-time student and teaching assistant (TA). I met with my TA supervisor Tom Pullum and notified him of my new diagnosis. We had no changes to make but I wanted to let Tom know that I could no longer drive in the state of Texas. We worked out plans if I happened to experience serious seizures during my computer labs. I notified my classmates and the Co-director of my dissertation. This was going to be a busy year and I was not going to let seizures stop my progress. I endured.

I had four of them today—bad kind. Had one while in French class and one while teaching stats lab. Had headaches all day today and last night—cuz of all these seizures (May 7, 1992).

This was a very productive year. I finished all necessary classes, began background work on my dissertation, chose my dissertation committee, took comprehensive examinations, and continued working as a counselor.

Counselor

I arrived in Austin late August 1991 as an epileptic. Once set up at University of Texas I scheduled an appointment with my supervisor at Child and Family Services (CFS) to discuss my seizures. I wanted to remain a part-time Counselor at CFS but my schedule would need to be altered. I no longer drove and thus followed public bus schedules on a daily basis. Sally and I talked for approximately an hour. My schedule was set up based on my needs. Never did we discuss my not returning as a Counselor. Several counselors/support staff arranged times to pick me up or drop me off at home and the University Campus. I rearranged times based on transportation—not based on my new seizures.

It was such a long day—I had a class, taught stats lab, and saw a few clients at CFS [Child and Family Services]. I had a pretty bad seizure on the bus tonight on the way home. I got off at the wrong bus stop—pretty far south from campus. It was a long walk. Pretty dark and quiet (February of 1992).

Many friends and colleagues were amazed that I continued to be a full time student and work as a Counselor after receiving "epilepsy" as a diagnosis. I don't think people realized I had been experiencing seizures for over ten years and continued to accomplish a great deal. This was a new time, however. I no longer had "feelings"—I was an epileptic.

All staff members were aware of my medical condition and I notified most of my clients. I had several seizures during sessions with clients. Most of these seizures seemed to be small. Thus, I could continue cognitive interaction with my clients. I do remember experiencing a few severe seizures. At this time I had a hand gesture which indicated I could not communicate with clients. When this happened the session would cease until I could once again interact with my client.

As I look back at this time period, I offered more to my clients than I ever expected. Many clients used me as a mentor. I endured seizures and continued full time as a student and part time as a counselor. I did not let my disability stop me from achieving my goals. I was an inspiration to my clients. As I look back at this time period, I was an inspiration to myself. I never quit.

Comprehensive Examinations

Most doctoral programs require passing "Comprehensive Examinations" before a doctoral student can be admitted to "candidacy." At the University of Texas—Austin, Comprehensive Exams are composed by three members of the particular Department. For me that was Sociology. My key area was "historical-comparative research methods." Every student chose an area of expertise and three faculty members developed an eight hour written exam. Most Committees offer a student a choice—two 4 hour tests or one 8 hour test. My Committee asked me to choose between one 8 hour test or a 6 hour test and a 2 hour test. I chose (to their preference) one 8 hour test. This was scheduled for October 1, 1991. The exam would start at 8:00 a.m., allow one hour for lunch, and end at 5:00 p.m. I studied for those exams for four months. I knew, however, that I had a barrier—I never knew exactly when I would seize.

> It's 10:30 p.m.—Comps are tomorrow—I wanted to write some now. I'm bouncing off the walls. I had a seizure today while talking to Dana about something—comps I'm sure—I don't know. I feel ok—I think. I am now in a different space. I'll write more tomorrow—I can do this (September 30, 1991).

I believe most students studied much of the night before comprehensive exams (maybe all night long—"all-nighters)." I didn't—I knew I had to sleep as much as possible. I knew my seizure threshold was lower if I went without sleep. I went to bed at 10:30 p.m. and woke up at 6:30 the next morning. I imagine most students fear comprehensive exams—if a student fails comps he/she can not advance into candidacy. I also had fears. I didn't fear "failing"—I feared seizures.

> It's 6:30 a.m.—Comps later. I have to write now and note my thoughts. I have such fears. What if I can't get to the test? What if I fall down the stairs? What if I seize during the test? I'll do it—I know I'll do good today. I'll write later.

I was set up in a private office on a desk top computer. I was to type all answers on "A" drive discs. I was nervous—not because of the material. I feared seizures. Because of this fear, I consistently saved all material I typed—probably every paragraph or so. Good idea. I did have a significant complex partial seizure (maybe a small one as well) during the test. I couldn't think for awhile and was quite nauseous. I could not understand English and was not quite sure where I was or what I should do. I certainly did not know how to use the computer. As the seizure began I got up and walked away from the computer and sat on a couch in the office. I knew I should be totally away from the desk or I might make serious mistakes on the computer at the peak of the seizure. As I recovered from the seizure I took in deep breaths. I had a headache. But I didn't leave the room or tell the proctor that I seized. I stopped writing for awhile (at least twenty minutes) and re-read my question and partial answer. I then started writing answers once again. That test had seven questions: six 1 hour questions and one 2 hour question. After recovery I kept pressing my mind until I was able to retrieve all my information. I endured. I never let the seizure(s) allow me to fail the test. I used the entire eight hours. The proctor came into the office to request the exam just as I was finishing. I had a chance to review all my answers—I was quite pleased with my capability to successfully finish the test. My brain was tired that night—from the seizure and the test. But I was happy—I passed through the right of passage. For a week I didn't even care if I failed—I finished the exam.

> 10:25 p.m.—Well, I did it—quite an experience. I had a seizure or two while taking comps—like couldn't understand the questions—so had to stop for awhile twice. I guess this is a "right of passage." Felt nausea for awhile but got done—I think ok (October 1, 1991).

I waited two weeks for the results of this exam. Finally, I asked a friend (Beth Gill) of mine what I should do to find out the results. Beth had taken a similar test (same Committee) over a year earlier. Great friend that she was, she contacted the Chair of the Committee. Dr. Sjoberg apologized for not notifying me—I did quite well on the exam and I was a Doctoral Candidate. It was time to start my Dissertation.

Dissertation

I began in-depth research for my dissertation after comprehensive exams in October of 1991. I was well aware that I was seizing regularly. I began adjusting my lifestyle to manage consistent seizures while conducting research for my dissertation.

The chair of my dissertation committee (Gideon Sjoberg) viewed the dissertation in a very broad prospectus. His questions were consistently based on the "mission" of the research project—the overall mission. Thus, he pushed for broad project goals—macro oriented. As much as I admired his style I could not work in this world. If I was going to obtain a Ph.D. while consistently experiencing seizures and negative side-effects of medications I had to push my stronger quality: micro managing.

Proposal

The Department of Sociology at the University of Texas requires a "proposal defense" before a candidate can begin the dissertation. Candidates are to conduct preliminary research on the research topic and present results to the

Committee. Committee members need to be convinced that the research question is valid and data is available. My defense was going to take place sometime in May of 1992.

When possible, I worked daily on my proposal. Because of seizures and medication I found that all days were not possible. However, consistent daily work schedules were usually possible. I called Sjoberg on a weekly basis to discuss progress. During these conversations, Sjoberg wanted to discuss data sources and progress on the research question. Sjoberg wanted me to set aside certain times on a certain day each week. I had to lie to him. I could not choose a specific day each week to work only on my proposal. I could not choose this time: my seizures chose the time I could work on the proposal. I worked on bits and pieces of the proposal every day when capable. When I called him weekly I had to pull all the pieces together to create the "vision" of the dissertation—convincing him that I had worked twenty-four hours the day before as instructed.

At the beginning of May Sjoberg was convinced I was ready to defend my proposal to my committee. I found a few hours that all members of the Committee could accept on May 15, 1992 and the room was selected. I had a seizure the night before the defense and the morning of the defense. Neither of these stopped me from defending my proposal.

> 5:20 p.m.—had one that left me tired (few almost or small ones too), felt like left body. Made me feel a little tired (May 14, 1992).

> 9 a.m.—Had a short one while brushing teeth [preparing for defense] (May 15, 1992).

I successfully defended my proposal the afternoon of May 15, 1992. I was able to once again combine all my bits and pieces as a mission for my dissertation. My Committee was convinced that I had the foundation for my research project. I was ready for the next step. I did not have a seizure during the defense but I had one right after it was over.

> 4:50 p.m.—[had seizure]—pretty disoriented—hated it. Well defense over— on my way to meet Sally et al [friends at outpatient clinic where I counseled] to celebrate. I drink a toast today—successful defense, the greatest Committee available and control of all that negative stuff—seizures et al (May 15, 1992).

These seizures did not stop me from celebrating with my friends at the Child and Family Services (CFS) where I was a part-time Counselor. I had a wonderful time with my friends that evening—headaches and all. I was ready to begin my dissertation.

Defense of Dissertation—August 2, 1994

I worked consistently on my dissertation from May 15, 1992 to August 2, 1994. Dr. Ronnelle Paulsen was appointed as co-director of my dissertation in 1992. This was a key offer by my Committee. Ronnelle was great at micro management. This was what I needed. It was necessary for me to contact Sjoberg every few weeks to review research progress—broad steps that responded to the research question, hurdles, and goals. On a daily basis I met with Ronnelle to discuss details. I was able to break broad goals down into small pieces with daily schedules and discussions.

During these two years I was experiencing at least thirty seizures a month, teaching a statistics lab, working as a therapist, and working on my dissertation. I needed to accomplish many small daily tasks on my dissertation if I was going to graduate in 1994. I would have failed if I remained in Sjoberg's "ballpark": only broad projects. In fact, many students did not survive the doctoral program. Many students dropped out before comprehensive exams. If students survived comprehensive exams, many drop out during the dissertation stage. Overall, many of Soberg's students did not graduate. I did not want this to happen. Through Ronnelle, I set up a very tight regimented schedule to continue progress on my dissertation.

During the year 1992–1993 I successfully conducted background research for my dissertation. I worked daily and consulted Paulsen regularly. During the year 1993–1994 I analyzed data and drew conclusions. I was also on the job market and sent out several applications each month. I interviewed for three faculty positions and accepted one in Raleigh, North Carolina in May of 1994.

The summer of 1994 was a very busy period. I had to prepare to move to Raleigh, NC at the beginning of August 1994. I had to defend my dissertation before leaving. I had to develop syllabi for four courses I would be teaching during the Fall of 1994. I believe I worked over twelve hours each day possible on my dissertation. On several occasions I spent hours (late at night on the phone) with my dissertation director Gideon Sjoberg. Finally, in July we agreed to arrange the dissertation defense. I would present my dissertation results to my entire Committee and answer any questions. This was called the "dissertation defense." The date was scheduled for the morning of August 2 of 1994. I experienced 33 seizures in July of 1994 (medium and bad type). The night before the dissertation I experienced one seizure (August 1, 1994). I did remain seizure-free during the defense. Only one Committee member was aware of my condition (Ronnelle Paulsen) and she had seen several of my episodes. As I entered that meeting I did not worry about my ability to intellectually defend my dissertation. I worried about seizures—would I be unable to defend the dissertation if I seized?

I remained seizure-free that day and successfully defended my dissertation. I obtained my Ph.D. My partner, Linda Tarkowski, had arranged a defense party for me in downtown Austin. I was able to walk into that room as Dr. Glumm. All my friends drank champagne in my honor.

Full-time Faculty

I moved to Raleigh, NC the day after my dissertation defense. I was beginning a new stage of my life: full-time faculty member at a four year college. I never told anyone at the school that I experienced seizures—at first. This did not stay a secret very long. After several weeks during my first semester I experienced an intense complex partial while lecturing. I could no longer communicate and thus could not describe my seizure to my students. After an hour of recovery I was able to describe my seizure condition to my colleagues.

My first four years at the College seemed to go well—seizures and all. I developed nine different courses. I usually taught four different courses per semester (most faculty only teach three different). I sat on several faculty/student Committees and was able to continue research. I had one article accepted for publication and had two others in process. I believe I was happy as possible. I did experience thirty or more seizures per month but I did not consider alternatives. I continued to stay on Tegretol and worked as hard as possible. As I look back as this time period, somewhere inside I knew negative changes were going to occur—I just didn't know when or how to handle the increased seizures.

SEIZURES INCREASE IN INTENSITY 1998—2001

My life began to change early in 1998. I set New Year's resolutions on January 3, 1998 without quite realizing the change in my seizure patterns. Thus, I did not realize how my life was going to change.

Car Accident—Retired Driver's License

I remember that January 23, 1998 was a difficult day. I had several severe complex partial seizures in the late morning. As a result of these seizures and intense headaches I decided to leave campus earlier than usual. While driving home I experienced another severe complex partial seizure. I remember the seizure starting and I knew it was going to be bad. The next thing I remember is someone knocking on my car window wondering if I was feeling okay.

I felt confused but okay. Suddenly I noticed my car was up against a tree. My chest was sore and my front window was cracked. I was able to get out of the car. Two men saw the accident and thus called the police. I was quite lucky. I did not hit another car and physically I was okay. I ruined my car that day. That seemed okay since I knew I could no longer safely drive.

I was sore for weeks and I had to change my life once again. I had to change my schedule. I found friends willing to pick me up and take me home. I became accustomed to the city bus schedules. However, I continued to work full-time and live my life as best as possible.

GRAND MAL SEIZURES

My seizure intensity continued to increase in 1998. I had a grand mal (generalized) seizure in my office on April 14, 1998. This was the first grand mal I experienced since 1991. I seized while continuing medications. This indicated I needed additional medications. This was when Depakote was added to my regimen. Once again my life changed. I was taking two medications: Depakote and Tegretol. I didn't drive. I experienced severe side-effects from Depakote and I continued experiencing at least 30 complex partial seizures each month. I think at this time I began withdrawing my society. I had a full-time job and I was a full-time epileptic.

Seizure intensity continued to increase even though I was taking two anti-epileptic medications. On September 23, 1999 I once again experienced a grand mal seizure in my office. At this time I needed to seek a new neurologist. After the school year I started seeing a University of North Carolina neurologist. A new medication was added to my regimen: Keppra. I was now on three medications continuing to experiencing 30—90 seizures each month. I continued to endure. I did have some inner anger at my brain. However, I buried this deep. So deep I didn't even realize this anger. I continue feeling denial—each seizure was going to be the last. I continued to bargain: I'll take drugs and sleep to quiet the brain. And, indeed, I was depressed. I was having trouble treating seizures.

Building Walls

During the 1998—1999 school year I began to change. I began building walls—separating myself from others. I spent more time at home. I met all goals at my college, continued research, and coped with seizures. However, I did not make many new friends. I kept most old friendships but only had new acquaintances. I guess I did not want to have to describe my condition to new close friendships. I did not know how to explain my condition to myself. I tried to "mask" limitations. My memory was beginning to weaken. Thus, I began learning planned responses to questions and I kept daily notes on what I did and what I should do next. I did not make as many plans for the future. I tried to deal with each day to the best of my ability. I was pulling away—from myself and others. As I look back from 1998—2001 my emotions were very "tight." I didn't express my true feelings. If I did, I would have to acknowledge fear and anger. So I "bottled" up my feelings. I continued taking medications, denied seizures would continue, and did not express true emotions.

Geographical Escape

During the 1998—1999 school I began looking for academic positions in Texas. As I look back on this time I was attempting a "geographical escape." I thought I wanted to return to Texas as a Faculty member of a Department of Sociology. I began searching for potential teaching positions in a variety of colleges in Texas. I had support from many friends on campus. I had letters of reference/recommendation prepared. I applied for several jobs in Texas and was interviewed by two. Both of these jobs were forced to close my potential position in the spring of 2000 due to budget weaknesses. I began searching for a new neurologist during 2000—2001 and still sent applications to a few colleges in Texas. I was convinced I wanted to return to this state. I don't think this was true. I think I wanted to return to a state where I lived not knowing I was an epileptic. I had two choices: Illinois and Texas. I think I wanted to run away from seizures—move to Texas and leave my seizure brain in Raleigh, NC. I was trying to escape.

There was no way I could escape my seizures. That chunk of my brain would have returned with me to Texas. At this time I knew I would have to seek a new neurologist and contemplate alternatives.

BENEFITS OF HISTORY AS CHILD OF AN ALCOHOLIC AND TORTURED OPTIMIST

As I look back, I endured seizures for over twenty-five years. Approximately four years before surgery, seizures became more frequent and intense: up to ninety per month. I never gave up hope. I dealt with a stigma and had endurance. I believe I coped with this condition and the social stigma because of my experience as a child of an alcoholic.

Stigma

Epilepsy is still associated with stigma in our society. Even today, people with epilepsy are incorrectly assumed to be far less intelligent than others or less able to hold a job. Self-stigma, in turn, results when the person with epilepsy begins to see herself in this same inaccurate light (Epilepsy Foundation 2001). The triple problem of medication side effects, personal fear of losing control, and society's revulsion of seeing a person struggle with a seizure add up to significant social barriers (Leppik 2000).

Diligence

According to my neurologist, Kevan VanLandingham, I was a very compliant patient. I had consistently attempted four different medications over ten years to control seizures. I never forgot to take my doses and never doubted the presence of my condition. All seizure medications have unpleasant side-effects. I experienced all of these. I had double vision from Tegretol. I experienced acute nausea from Depakote. Keppra added to nausea when taken with Tegretol. Dilantin may cause facial hair. I never complained about the side effects. I grew up in a dysfunctional family and learned tolerance and endurance. I also followed the rules given by "authority figures" (which would include neurologists). I believe these experiences helped me cope with seizures. I never complained about seizures or medication side effects, and I never "gave up." I accepted my diagnosis—just as I accepted the conditions of my family. I figured seizures were just a part of my body. My neurosurgeon, Michael Haglund, has known, treated, hundreds of people with epilepsy. But he argues I was different. The degree to which I functioned amazed him. By the time I became Haglund's patient in 2001 I had been a faculty member of a local College for seven years. I had published articles in academic journals, and was working on a book about the way organizations construct markets for products and services in mental health. Haglund had never known a patient with the fortitude to accomplish what I had managed having 30 or 40 seizures a month.

> If you pick the range of epilepsy patients and what they do, a lot of them are on disability." "A lot of them are working at lower-paying jobs. Not too many of them have doctoral degrees. I mean, that's just a credit to her and her motivation and inner strength to push through even though she was being tortured all the time by these seizures and not knowing when it's going to happen" (Miller 2002).

As I look back on this time period, I endured seizures and coped with stigma and discrimination because I learned endurance as a child of an alcoholic. I also am a "tortured optimist." I always thought the seizures would decrease and eventually disappear. I believe this experience was important. In fact, perhaps I should have complained sooner. Sometimes I believe I coped with seizures and side effects too long. However, this is all hindsight. Perhaps, in come strange way, my anger regarding my condition and treatment is what inspired me to seek a new neurologist to consider alternative treatment.

Chapter Four

Challenging the Spirit
5/1/2001–Fall of 2001

Illness as Metaphor:
"Illness is the night-side of life
Everyone who is born holds dual citizenship:
In the kingdom of the well and the kingdom of the sick
Although we prefer to use only the good passport
Sooner or later each of us is obliged to identify ourselves
As citizens of that other place"

Susan Sontag (1978)

BACKGROUND

Significant changes in my seizure patterns began during the 1998–1999 school year. Seizures increased in frequency and intensity and medications no longer offered reasonable protection. I experienced two grad mal seizures and several hundred severe partial seizures during this academic year. Linda Tarkowski (clinical pharmacist) and a neurologist indicated that over time Tegretol (my primary anti-convulsant) seemed to weaken. A new medication (Depakote) was added to my drug regimen. This medication did not offer enough support. Seizures continued to increase in intensity. At this time I began seeing another neurologist at University of North Carolina—Chapel Hill. A new medication was added—Keppra. However, this medication did not seem to offer significant protection. The academic years of 1999–2000 and 2000–2001 were difficult academic years. Seizures continued. Alternative treatment seemed necessary. Medications were not controlling seizures. In May of 2001 I (with advice) decided it was time to seek a new neurologist. At this time I was taking three medications but continued to seizure on a regular basis. I was referred to Duke Hospital for alternative testing and intervention. In late spring 2001 I, for the first time, met my neurologist Dr. Kevan VanLandingham.

ENTER DUKE ASSESSMENT: KEVAN VANLANDINGHAM

What does it take to inspire investigation or change?
Sheldon Ekland-Olson

I met Dr. Kevan VanLandingham for the first visit on May 24, 2001. After reviewing my case he encouraged in-depth testing to locate the seizure focal point and determine if removal was possible. With caution, I agreed to the testing.

The First Step of Recovery for Adult Children of Alcoholics
(www.geocities.com/howitworks2001/)
We acknowledge and accept that we are powerless in controlling the lives of self or others, and that trying to control self/others makes our lives unmanageable.

Medical Testing

I entered Duke Hospital (Durham, NC) for clinical testing on July 2, 2001. Dr. Kevan VanLandingham planned to conduct a series of tests to locate the seizure focal point. Once located, tests would be conducted to determine if removal was possible. During the previous ten years I had been tested many times but the focal point was never determined. Dr. VanLandingham had a new plan. In order to locate the focal point, I needed to experience a range of seizures under surveillance.

Upon intake I stopped taking all anti-seizure medications and was hooked up to a twenty-four hour EEG to attempt to locate the focal point when I experienced seizures. Dr. VanLandingham was interested in a series of seizures to ensure I had only one focal point. He encouraged me to stay awake for at least twenty-four hours. A "sleep-deprived" brain tends to have a much lower seizure threshold. I would be lying in bed for several days and awake for the first twenty-four hours.

I was closely monitored during the testing period. I was under twenty-four hour surveillance by a camera. If I walked around the room the camera would follow me. Medical practitioners wanted to observe all physical movements during seizures several times to search for patterns. I was on a cardiac monitor during this time period and was hooked up to a twenty-four hour EEG.

Thus, the cords were long enough that I could walk around that small room. I could use the restroom but no shower for several days. Medical staff took my vital signs every two hours: blood pressure, temperature, and pulse (even though I was hooked up to the cardiac monitor). The vein on my left arm was ready to accept medications if necessary. After I had a series of seizures I would be injected with valium to quiet the brain and reduce the chance of seizures.

My "wish list" was strange during this time period. For the first time in my life I "hoped" I would have a series of seizures. I was off medications for at least two days and had been awake for twenty-four hours straight before I had my first severe complex partial seizure. Over the next few days I experienced three more severe complex partial seizures. I do not have a clear memory of these seizures (this indicates they were very serious complex partials). I do remember recovering from the seizures. Nursing staff would enter my room and begin to ask questions. I was asked what time of day it was, what specific date it was, and what particular objects were (for example, a nurse would point to her watch and ask me what was the object). I had difficulty understanding the questions or providing answers for a significant period of time (twenty minutes to an hour). I remember telling a nurse the year was 1999 (correct year 2001) and that the President was Bill Clinton (correct answer Bush). I have wondered if I was really confused after the serious seizure or if I wished it WAS 1999 with Bill Clinton president. I was able to acknowledge that the nurse was pointing to her "watch." However, I could not detect the face, band, or hands of the watch. This indicated a long "post-ictil" or recovery stage: I had trouble with memory, accuracy, and details. I remember watching these seizures on film from the camera placed in my room. For the first time in my life I was able to watch myself experience a series of seizures. It was at this time that Dr. Kevan VanLandingham felt four seizures offered enough data to locate the seizure focal point. I only had one focal point. This was a positive find. A brain with a series of focal points is not an appropriate candidate for surgical removal at this point in time.

WADA

After testing, Kevan told me the seizure focal point was located in my dominant left temporal lobe. I needed a new test: WADA. This was a test developed by a female practitioner to determine the strength of each lobe independently. Twice I was injected with an anesthetic. My right lobe was tested first with the left lobe asleep. I wasn't able to speak, felt sedated, and I had double-vision. Thus I had some difficulty with the test. However, I was able to remember most of the pictures I was shown. Next, my left lobe was tested with my right asleep. I did not even feel the anesthetic. I did not have double-vision and I could speak just fine. I was able to answer all questions on the test. According to Kevan, my left lobe was dominant but my right lobe was strong enough. Thus, removal of part of my left lobe was now acceptable. My brain would remain strong enough post surgery.

Decision For Surgery

"Critical moments can make discourse on an issue visible as they stimulate commentary"

William Gamson (1992)

I remember the moment I decided to undergo neurosurgery. According to VanLandingham and Haglund (neurosurgeon), I had "passed" all the tests and was determined to be an appropriate surgical candidate. I had to make a final decision: was it worth it? I have these seizures but are they so bad that I must endure neurosurgery? Can I handle recovery? What are the side effects? Will I die on the table? Will I be further disabled after surgery? I was still in a state of denial and I was scared. I did believe in a higher power as a child of an alcoholic. However, I still did not admit I was powerless over seizures or accept a "higher power" as an epileptic. I did not feel "hope" and did not feel "worthy" of the surgery. I did have other emotions. I believe fear was trumped by another emotion: anger. I was so angry at Meredith College and I wanted to fight back but could not unless I was stronger (i.e. less seizures, stronger brain). I couldn't support my claim that I endured discrimination until I was strong enough to fight in court. I was so angry that I could endure surgery. I signed the forms and agreed to surgery.

I knew surgery was not scheduled until August. Thus, I had a few weeks to "rethink" my decision. I can't remember the exact date, but finally, in late July 2001 I accepted the COA first step as an epileptic. Surgery was an appropriate step or my life would remain unmanageable. I didn't realize it at the time, but I began adopting the COA twelve step recovery program. I once again took the first step: the most difficult. This time I was honest. I was powerless over seizures and my life had become unmanageable.

NEUROSURGERY: MICHAEL HAGLUND

The Second and Third Steps of Recovery for Adult Children of Alcoholics
(www.geocities.com/howitworks2001/)
We have come to believe that a power greater than ourselves can restore enough order and hope in our lives to move us to a growth framework.

We make the decision to turn our lives over to this power to the best of our ability, and honestly accept that taking responsibility for ourselves is the only way growth is possible.

I was a member of a specific group of patients. I developed this concept while researching patients in 1994. I called this group the "privileged vulnerable."

Privileged Vulnerable

This group possesses a set of resources that are not always available to other vulnerable groups. This group may be acutely and temporarily impaired (physical complications, suicidal, depressed, or other trouble managing their lives) and thus is vulnerable. However, this group possesses a set of personal and social resources (friends, family, physicians, attorneys) that aid them in their attempts to fight back against exploitation. This group is fairly sophisticated and thus possesses knowledge of hospital and court bureaucracies (Glumm 1994).

I believe I was a member of the privileged vulnerable. I was a vulnerable medical patient. I was experiencing 30–90 seizures per month and was contemplating neurosurgery. However, I was privileged. I was a full-time employee and thus have strong health insurance coverage. I was educated. I have a Ph.D. in the field of Sociology. I also have experience with medical treatment. I was a social service worker for ten years and thus knew the "language" of the field. I had enormous support from friends and family. A close friend had a Clinical Doctoral degree in a medical field. Thus I had an advocate to assess my case and offer support as I considered surgery.

Surgery

I checked into Duke Hospital on August 14, 2001. I did not realize this at the time, but upon check-in, I took the next two steps in my twelve step recovery program. I believed that a "power" greater than me could restore order in my life. I made a decision to turn my life over to this higher power and I accepted full responsibility for all decisions in my life. For the first time in over twenty-five years I was relaxed. I accepted myself as an epileptic and believed order was to be restored in my life.

Surgery was scheduled for the next day. Preparations began August 14, 2001. I remember waking up on the morning of August 15, 2001. It was a strange experience. This could be the last day of my life. Or, it could be the first day of a new, stronger, happier, and more fulfilling life. I was not able to eat (because of surgical anesthetics). Perhaps this was a benefit—I did not have to face the "last meal" impression. I was prepped for surgery late morning. I remember receiving pre-surgical testing (to ensure I was ready) and eventually taking medications. Surgery (according to Linda) began about 2:00 p.m. I don't remember much of this time period (as a result of brain surgery and complications). What I do remember and what spaces I can fill in are valuable.

I thought I would "sleep" through surgery. However, this did not happen. The seizures were located in my left brain hemisphere. I am right handed and thus left brain dominant. The "broca" is located in the dominant lobe. The broca houses "speech" and thus can not be removed. The surgeons knew where the origin of the seizures was located but did not know where the broca was or what "brain activities" were connected to the seizure focal point. Thus the surgeons wanted to "map" my brain—figure out which part of the brain controlled speech and which part controlled movement. While performing surgery on my left brain lobe the surgeons woke me up several times to search for the broca. I was shown many pictures and asked many questions. I was asked to move my arms and legs, blink my eyes, and answer questions. Eventually, I was not able to answer questions. I believe I heard someone say "we've got it." Speech was located and was far enough away from the origin of the seizures—thus removal of the focal point could begin. I don't remember much after that. Apparently I was able to convey a message to Linda through medical support staff. I told her to say "hi chabba" on my behalf. Surgery was finished at approximately 10:30 p.m. (on August 15, 2001) and I was transferred to ICU for the initial stage of recovery.

Survival

I survived surgery. However, it seems others thought survival was questionable. Apparently I slipped into a coma twice. Others thought I might die in the hospital.

Apparently I did well in the initial stage of recovery: the first twenty-four hours after surgery. At approximately 5:00 p.m. on August 16 I was transferred from ICU to a room in Duke Hospital. I seemed to do well for the next twenty hours. However, I started losing ground at 1:00 p.m. on August 17. I don't remember this at all. My brain was quite swollen and I was having trouble answering questions. By 5:00 p.m. Linda noticed my eyes were glazed and I was losing consciousness. By 6:00 p.m. Dr. Haglund sent me for a CT scan and increased medications. This was a difficult evening. I had trouble breathing and was never quite comfortable. I vaguely remember pain, fear, and discomfort. I was transferred to ICU once again the morning of August

18, 2001. I believe I slipped in and out of consciousness several times. I was unconscious much of the time and having several motor seizures the morning of August 19. Thus, medical staff increased intervention. It was decided (by support and medical staff) to intubate me and start a Versed drip. This heavy medication was to "relax brain"—hence my first coma.

I spent a few days in intensive care. I vaguely remember waking up in restraints a few times. According to Linda Tarkowski, I had tried to pull at bandages on my head several times so I was placed in restraints. I was extubated Tuesday morning—I don't remember this. When I woke up I felt pain. I couldn't talk and didn't know how to self-induce morphine. I am very grateful that Linda (close friend) was there and she could tell by my eyes and gestures that I was feeling pain and thus she gave me a hit of morphine. I remember the pain dissipating. However, I would feel my face itching (side-effect of morphine). I could not reach my face because of the restraints. I also could not speak so I couldn't tell others my face was itchy. I just tried to sleep as much as possible but I could never sleep for a long period of time due to discomfort. I was never comfortable and always tried to move around in bed (seeking relaxation). For a few days I didn't/couldn't relax at all. Every memory I have at this time is based on fear and discomfort.

I significantly improved on August 23, 2001. I was transferred to step-down care. This I do remember. I didn't like transfers—I liked staying in the same room. I also needed to be transferred in the hospital for several tests (CAT scans and MRIs to record brain activity). I didn't like the testing either. I believe I was uncomfortable being moved (brain was sensitive and I always felt cold and uncomfortable). I believe I was also afraid of change—I had a difficult time learning where I was and thus did not like to be moved.

Two days later (August 25) I spent time with my first speech pathologist. I was asked many questions regarding day/time/events/memories. I struggled on this exam. I had difficulty remembering the date or how old I was. I knew I was at Duke Hospital but I thought this hospital was in Duke, North Carolina (actually Durham, North Carolina). The therapist knew I was not ready for discharge. I was not able to verbally communicate my needs or wishes. Thus, self-care was questioned. I remember this time period. I knew when I needed food or fluids and I knew how to get them in my home. However, language was weak and thus I could not verbally communicate my plan. I was advised to seek speech therapy after discharge. I agreed.

Later that same day it seems I began to fail once again. According to Linda, it seems my behavior suddenly became erratic. I must press that it is necessary to have a family member or close friends with you during surgery recovery. Significant others will notice a significant change in behavior (professionals will not be as aware). I don't remember this experience, but apparently I left my bed to use the restroom. Linda knows I wash my hands after using the restroom on a regular basis. In fact I have been a bit compulsive in this area. I have always washed my hands after everything (to minimize infections, flu symptoms). This set off an alarm in Linda. I don't remember, but she asked if I was feeling ok. I didn't answer the question. This encouraged Linda to look in my eyes and check temperature. Apparently, Linda saw I experienced an altered mental status (poor eye contact) and felt "warm" to touch. I had a fever and began to slip off into another coma. Linda called in medical professionals and had to convince them that the fever was not the only symptom. Fever seems to be a normal side effect to surgery and thus medical staff were not concerned. Linda was. Most patients can tolerate a low-grade fever but I just had brain surgery and thus a portion of my skull was removed and my brain vulnerable. My behavior was erratic and my eyes suggested altered mental status. Linda encouraged the resident to continue testing and contact Dr. Michael Haglund. Eventually, it was determined that I had a severe infection on my arm—central line of medications. The central line was moved into a new vein. The infection was treated with antibiotics. I had a few tough days and was unconscious most of the time. I remember waking up several times. I remember hallucinations as a result of the fever. I saw money flying around the room. Linda asked if I thought the money was "really there." I told her "no, but I see it." I knew this hallucination was a result of the fever. The next time I woke up I was packed in ice. I was hot, hurting, and freezing at the same time. Many times I would begin to sweat as a result of the fever. This encouraged the heart monitor to begin beeping. I woke up a few times to the heart monitor. Interestingly, nurses seemed to ignore the monitor many times. Linda (when available) was able to reset the monitor. I remember the monitor beeping a few times when Linda was not in the room. I had to contact nurses (via call button) several times before visited. I had difficulty breathing several days and thus was once again placed on a respirator. I remember waking up once again and feeling the tube in my lungs. Many times I felt alone in the room (if Linda was not present) during this time—and afraid. I didn't trust certain nurses. Many nurses (i.e. Owen) were fantastic and I felt calmer when they were on staff. This I remember well—I slept better when Owen (RN) was down the hall.

Recovery improved significantly, once again, on August 27, 2001. I was, once again, going to be extubated. This I remember. As uncomfortable as the tube in the lungs might seem, my greatest fear was removal of this tube. I have watched so many medical shows on television and it has always seemed that the removal of this tube was uncomfortable and painful. As a child of an alcoholic I always "imagine" an event feeling worse than it will. This again happened with the respirator. The removal of that tube did not even feel uncomfortable. I think the hours of dreading this removal was far worse than the event itself. I continued recovering well that day. Late that night I realized this had been the first seizure-free day of most of my life.

The two weeks in the hospital were troubling, frightening, and painful. However, I must press that they were not nearly as bad as my twenty-five years experience with continued seizures. According to neurologists, medical staff, and my neurosurgeon, my stay in the hospital was more difficult than "average" for invasive surgery. However, for me, my experience was well worth it. My acceptance of powerless and belief in a higher power helped me start a new life. My diligence as a recovering COA helped me endure.

Discharge

I believe my last seizure was August 26, 2001. During initial recovery I experienced several different types of seizures—mostly motor seizures. My mouth or hands might jerk for several minutes. This type of seizure might be common for anyone experiencing brain surgery. Seizure-free time began 8/27/2001.

During the next few days recovery was smooth. The feeding tube was removed and I was able to begin eating hospital food again (unpleasant as the food was I realized this was a positive experience). My neurologist and neurosurgeon were discussing discharge. I knew who I was, where I was, how old I was, and who was president. I helped set some plans for recovery. Before I could be discharged, however, I had to learn to walk and learn to use the restroom on my own. This was a challenge. The catheter was removed and I went into the restroom. Once I sat in the restroom for an hour and finally I requested a catheter. Finally my nurse, Owen, removed the catheter and tried to teach me to use the restroom on my own. Once again, I sat in the restroom (failing) for an hour. Owen asked if he could come into the restroom. Why not, I am just sitting here doing nothing. He encouraged me to smell an alcohol swab. Wow, that was great. Finally, I did use the toilet and could request discharge from the hospital. I also learned to walk again. Nausea increased as I tried to leave the bed. I remember walking with support staff a few times. I was congratulated by several nurses in the hallway. I must admit that experiencing the hall was interesting. I felt, for the first time, that I had entered a new world. If not a seizure-free world—it was to be a "recovery" world. I was frightened but I was ready to leave this "treatment" world and enter "recovery."

I was discharged August 29, 2001. My sister arrived August 29 to stay with me for the first days of recovery. I remember crying when she entered my room. I am not sure why I cried. Was I learning how to once again express emotions? Had I feared I might never see her again? Was I mourning the past twenty years?

Recovery

I continued recovery after discharge from Duke Hospital Center. I still had a great deal to accomplish. I had difficulty walking, talking, and eating. I needed to be supervised twenty-four hours per day. I was afraid to be alone because I did not know how to follow directions. My partner and sister escorted me through the house, gave me medications, and provided food. I could not be trusted on my own.

My definition of "difficult" was derived from my history as a child of an alcoholic and a seizure-oriented lifestyle. As difficult as surgery and recovery seemed to others, they were nothing when compared to my twenty-five year seizure history.

Speech Therapy

As mentioned, I was encouraged to seek speech therapy after discharge. I had difficulty communicating with others on a consistent basis. I was always "searching" for words. Many times friends had to complete sentences for me. Dr. Michael Haglund referred me to a speech therapist upon discharge: Lina Karoukas at Wake Forest Rehabilitation. I was scheduled for an evaluation for September 4, 2001. I remember this day well. I was still in recovery. I had difficulty choosing appropriate words when speaking to others and Lina was aware of this quickly. At the end of the evaluation, she encouraged three appointments per week for the next six weeks. I knew at that time that I did not have the capability to attend three sessions per week. I didn't drive and thus needed friends to escort me to the appointments. Physically I did not have the endurance for three appointments per week. I agreed to two appointments per week and homework. Speech therapy began on September 20, 2001 (I had to wait almost three weeks for insurance approval). I was able to arrange transportation. Two friends agreed to drive me once per week. Liz Wolfinger offered to drive me on Mondays and Sam Carothers volunteered transport on Thursday. This fit my schedule well.

Of course this was called "speech therapy." However, I was learning how to exercise my brain: I was expanding neurological capabilities.

After the evaluation, I attended therapeutic sessions (forty-five minutes per session) five times and worked on homework assignments every night for three weeks. During each session Lina showed me pictures and I was to identify the object (i.e. funnel, hoop, football, toaster, ect). I was read two minute stories. I was then asked several questions regarding these stories to record my capability to understand the material. Many times events were described and I was to determine the schedule of the events and who performed which task. The best way to describe these sessions and homework assignments is "brain teasers." I was worried about these sessions for the first two weeks and feared homework assignments. I always wanted to be home alone when I did the homework. I kept working hard to increase brain activity. After several sessions it was determined I was much stronger. October 8, 2001 was my last session. During this session Lina compared my capabilities from the first session to this day. I had done well in less time than anticipated. I graduated from speech therapy on October 8, 2001. However, I continue "brain teasers" on a continual basis.

Progression

I needed consistent recovery upon discharge from Duke Hospital. I still felt pain, had difficulty eating, had trouble following orders (thus others monitored medications and actions), needed exercise, and speech therapy. I was still physically weak and thus my days were short for awhile. I woke up late in the morning, took a nap, and went to bed early in the evening. My brain was weak for a few weeks. Although I enjoyed talking with visitors and friends over the phone but I couldn't handle these interactions for any longer than an hour. Within a few weeks my day became longer. My appetite increased and I was able to exercise moderately (supervised walking). I was able to enjoy television shows, read the newspaper, and enjoy conversations for longer periods of time. This was less than two months from the day of the surgery. This was just the beginning of a life-long enthralling recovery.

RECOVERING

Following the philosophy of Alcoholics Anonymous, I am quite aware that I am not "recovered" from epilepsy. I will never be "cured" of epilepsy. Recovery is the process of bringing problems into a state of stable remission (White 2000). I am in the state of remission. I have not seized since August 26, 2001. I am in recovery—an ongoing process.

State of Recovery

Everyone has a seizure threshold. For most people, that level is very high. For most people a seizure may occur with a high fever, a brain tumor, spinal infections, dehydration, low electrolytes (sodium and sugar), hypoxia (low oxygen), excessive use of stimulants, withdrawal from sedative drugs, or massive sleep deprivation (Leppik 2000). Because I had a seizure focal point I had a much lower threshold. Many body changes inspired thirty to ninety seizures every month for years. As a result of this experience (even after removal of the focal point) I will always have a low seizure threshold. Therefore, I am not cured of epilepsy. I am recovering—I hope for a very long time. I will always be aware that I could experience a seizure as a result of some physical trauma. I am Karen Glumm, the Child of an Alcoholic with a history of seizures.

Adopting the Twelve Step Recovery Process for Adult Children of Alcoholics

During late fall of 2001 I realized I began adopting the COA twelve step recovery process as an epileptic in the summer of 2001. As hard as I had tried to manage seizures since 1991 I had never fully acknowledged that I was powerless. In the summer of 2001 I acknowledged that I was powerless in controlling the seizures and that my life was unmanageable. It was at this time that I had come to believe that a power greater than myself could restore enough order and hope in my life to move me to a growth framework. I made my decision to turn my life over to this power to the best of my ability and accept taking responsibility for myself in the only way growth was possible. For the first six months after surgery I continued to work the first three steps. I was in recovery—I had not seized for a few months. However, I was well aware that I could seize again and continued the twelve step recovery process. I celebrated the value of my past as a recovering child of an alcoholic. I learned patience, tolerance, and acceptance. I knew then that I would continue my twelve step program as a child of an alcoholic and an epileptic.

For those epileptics who are seizure-free (as a result of surgery or medications) or may still seize (as we all may), I encourage you to adopt the twelve-step recovery process. We are in recovery but we may still seize—relapse. Each morning I tell myself I am an epileptic and will continue recovery. I was seizure-free yesterday and am working on recovery today.

Chapter Five

Facing the Skeletons in the Closet[1]
Early Fall 2001

The Fourth Step of Recovery for Adult Children of Alcoholics
(www.geocities.com/howitworks2001/)
We make an inventory of ourselves, looking for our mental, optional, spiritual, physical, volitional and social assets and liabilities. We look at what we
have, how we use it, and how we can acquire what we need.

Part of recovery is to notice and successfully release the skeletons in the
closet. My closet has been so full that I have been unsuccessful storing personal belongings. For the first time in well over twenty-five years I am ready
to clean the closet. Let's meet and face the skeletons (at least those of which
I am aware).

IDENTIFYING THE SKELETONS

Seizures

The largest skeleton in the closet is a history of seizures. I have experienced
complex partial seizures[2] (irregularly) since I was a child. These began to occur regularly in the late 1970's. My thoughts and feelings seemed altered. Old
memories would flash through my mind (i.e. déjà vu). I would begin to sweat
(i.e. raise in blood pressure) and my pulse would begin to race. My memory
seemed impaired: I may not be totally convinced where I was, what time of
day it was, what I should be doing, and where I should be going. My mind
was "cloudy" and I always felt fear. Many times I could not understand language. I didn't know what was going to happen and how I could deal with
anything. I began calling this the "feeling" in the late 1970's.

In the summer of 1980, these "feelings" increased in frequency and intensity. I began to notice physical side effects: nausea, "cloudy mind," and impaired memory.

> Got up and went to work—day went fast—felt sick—didn't talk to many people. In the camera room I felt weird again—slowing me down. Weird feeling comes a lot—wonder what it means. I am sick of this "feeling"—will it destroy me (Summer 1980 personal journal)?

For the first time in my life I failed to show up for scheduled events. Many friends and colleagues believed this meant I "didn't care."

> Slept in—having such a hard time remembering things—can't stand it. Time is slipping away. Didn't feel like eating, thinking, anything because of "weird feeling." Lori [Steele] came over for awhile—Lori could see I was sick with "feeling." I feel something in me dying every day. Things get worse with every breath, every moment. I am in a terrible mood—"feeling" is getting me down—feel jail (Fall 1980 personal journal).

I didn't know how to explain my physical impairment. Criticism for "lack of dedication" seemed easier than explaining the "feelings." In fact, I tried to explain these "feelings" to several friends—only to be stared at with implied disbelief. In early 1981 I worked up courage to see three physicians. I described, to the attempt possible, my brain "feelings." Two physicians offered anti-depressants. The third offered a different medication: Ritalin. I was a graduate student and knew this medication was for attention deficit disorder. I was quite sure that my condition did not indicate depression or attention deficit and never accepted the prescriptions. I stopped telling others and endured my life for six months. During 1981 the frequency and intensity of episodes increased dramatically. I once again explained these to a close friend—Lori Steele—studying to become a medical/surgical nurse. For the first time someone listened. I still remember her response: "Karen, that sounds like a type of seizure." I went to our local library to read on types of seizures. In the early 1980's the only types of seizures written about frequently were grand mal and petit mal. Anyone experiencing these seizures seemed to lose total consciousness and never quite remember the event. This did not describe my seizures. Unfortunately, I always remember the embarrassing event. Several months later I began to work with the Coles County Association for Retarded Citizens (CCAR). I searched the medical journals available in this organization and no description diagnosed my "feeling" as a seizure. It was at this time I pushed the seizure skeleton deep into my closet. The "feeling" was once again a hidden secret and would remain in the back of that closet for ten years. I denied I even experienced these physical traumas —each one was going to be the "last." No friends or co-workers would ever know about my personality "quirks." Until 1991.

My personal journal does not discuss partial episodes between 1982– 1991—I accepted them as a "personality quirk"—a form of denial. 1981 was one of the most difficult years—until 1991.

I experienced my first Grand Mal (generalized) seizure on June 22, 1991. I was asked if I ever before experienced a Grand Mal seizure—of course I said no. I had not. After routine hospital testing (EEG, lumbar puncture, and CT scan) my seizure was diagnosed as idiopathic—no known cause. No prescriptions necessary. For awhile I believed this.

> I'm in Irving Hospital [Texas]— . . . I had a seizure . . . I have been here for 40 hours—had a CT and then a spinal puncture. . . On Dilantin now—hopefully temporary as they [physicians] rule stuff out. It is strange to have a [first] seizure at [age] 32 (personal journal).

Until July 13, 1991. I experienced another Grand Mal seizure—now a pattern. I was placed on medications and could not drive in the state of Texas for a year. My life was going to change—I was an epileptic.

> . . . I had another seizure this morning—6:00 a.m. My life is going to change now—will have to be on meds awhile and I may lose my license . . . I just can't believe this—seizures at 33—damn. It's hard to hope now—I'm seizure prone. I go back and forth—from being ok with this to being angry, sad, and afraid (personal journal).

I began to read more current medical research on epilepsy supplied by a friend. For the first time I noticed a new type of seizure: complex partial. In some ways the "feeling" skeleton came out of the closet at this time. The skeleton had a new name—epileptic. Now the "feeling" would be treatable with medication. However, the seizures never stopped. I kept adding medications and seizures increased in intensity and frequency. I could now tell friends and colleagues the name of the skeleton. Many accepted my condition and many supported. For awhile. I did have new restrictions. Grand mal seizures were in check but the complex partials continued so much so that the skeleton grew in size and needed to be shoved back into the closet. I desired to continue work in my doctoral program. I continued to work as a part-time therapist, gather and analyze data for my dissertation, and taught the Statistics lab for the Department of Sociology at University of Texas at Austin. I didn't have time for a disability—I was too busy and didn't like the social or medical interpretation. All I had was a minor inconvenience. Thirty to ninety seizures per month would not stop accomplishments and thus the skeleton remained deep in the closet. I still recorded every seizure. However, I continued to convince myself that each one was the last (a state of denial). Every seizure was a nail on the closet door—imprisoning the skeleton. Until the summer of 2001.

Memory Impairment

The next largest skeleton was memory losses. I lost a close friend in the early 1980's because I failed to show up for a few appointments. It was at this time that I first noticed memory impairment. In earlier years my memory was so strong. I had not accepted memory losses yet and failed to record engagements. I made promises—didn't record in a schedule—and failed to remember appointments because of seizures. I didn't know how to tell a friend that I broke a promise because of the "feeling." Instead, I apologized and said I "forgot." To many people that indicated that I didn't care. In the summer of 1981 this skeleton was created. Once again, 1980–1981 was one of the toughest years with frequency and intensity of seizures—until 1991. In 1982 I began keeping a consistent personal calendar—of appointments, chores, and accomplishments. I had never needed to record dates, phone numbers, or bills. It was at this time I failed to pay a few bills, forgot phone numbers, and forgot birthdays or anniversaries.

In the early 1990's the strength and length of the complex partials increased—this began to significantly affect memory. The skeleton increased in size. I shoved that thing as deep in the closet as possible—she kept bumping into the epileptic skeleton.

I began to keep in-depth notes—what did I do (every activity), what will I do, how did I complete a chore, what should I read, what did I read, who called, who should have called, who should I call, etc. I learned how to record behavior and events as a Social Service Worker—now I knew I had to record my own day in detail. A high percent of time would be spent on notes. Every night I would review what I did and what I would do the next day. Every morning I reviewed what I had done the day before and what I would do that day. The skeleton kept popping out of the closet—larger and larger. Memory impairment was embarrassing. I didn't know how to describe or live with this condition. I was forty years old with a memory becoming weaker every year. What would the future be like? Could I remember my past? Would I be able to remember where the "memory" skeleton was in the closet? Would I remember where the closet was? This skeleton was noticed by another one: fears skeleton.

Fears

For the first time in my life I can identify the fears. This list has grown over the past twenty-five years. Because of the seizures and these fears I was never completely relaxed: I was always nervous and on edge. I now know this list of fears grew because of the increased frequency and intensity of seizures. These fears have dissipated during recovery but I remember them well. Let's notice the fears and embrace these skeletons.

> Hard to get used to this—adjusting. My fears are there—lots of fears—of someone breaking in, raping me, something happening. I feel dependent. Couple of seizures today—one kinda bad and two after that one—felt fear of where I was (January 18, 1993 personal journal).

Being Alone

> It's so difficult being alone—I'm major dependent. Seizures have made this (July 13, 1993 personal journal).

I have experienced the fear of being alone for twenty years. I believe this fear appeared the same time as my first complex partial seizure. As a teenager I loved having the house to myself. Several times my parents and younger siblings went off on vacations and I had the house to myself. The "feelings" (seizures) developed during the 1979–1980 academic year and greatly increased during the 1980–1981 academic year. I had the house to myself for several weeks during the summer of 1980. For the first time in my life I felt fear as my family was leaving. I had difficulty relaxing or sleeping the first several days. I could never explain this response to being "alone." I now know I feared being in the house alone while experiencing seizures. What if the phone rang? What if someone was at the door? What if the stove was on? I ended up staying with my older brother for several nights and visiting friends on other nights.

This fear increased strongly during the next twenty years. I never lived alone or chose to stay alone. If roommates were traveling and I was alone I was nervous. That poor skeleton shook in the closet—even while sharing the space with others.

Lighting Candles

As much as I love candles, I began to fear lit candles if I was home alone. I now understand. I was afraid I would have a very severe partial seizure with lit candles. If I had a long recovery period there may have been a chance of a

fire in the house. This was always a possibility. I never lit a candle when I was
alone. When friends came over I lit candles immediately but remembered to
blow them out when I was once again alone.

Cooking/Use of Stove

In the late 1990's I began to fear use of the stove if I was in a house by myself. Seizure intensity increased dramatically. I remember seizing many times
while trying to cook or heat water in the kettle. If I anticipated a severe partial seizure with a difficult recovery period I tried to turn off the stove in advance. I was usually successful at turning off the stove. However, I remember several times I was not successful and thus burned food in the oven. Once
I experienced a severe partial seizure as the kettle began to whistle. I was not
able to respond and a friend rushed into the kitchen to turn off the stove. Once
I had a very severe complex partial (at least an hour of recovery). Twenty
minutes after the seizure I was trying to make coffee to ease a throbbing
headache (as a result of the severe complex partial seizure). I failed to grind
the beans and was using cold water. A friend came into the kitchen and offered her services for completing the coffee. I was able to leave the kitchen,
relax, and drink hot coffee a few minutes later.

> I had a bad seizure today. I wanted coffee but couldn't grind the beans or heat
> water. LT helped. God I hate this. My head still hurts and I couldn't think
> (Spring 1999 personal journal).

Until surgery in 2001 I never enjoyed cooking or using the stove. Until
now I could not have explained why. I no longer fear the use of the stove. I
never talked much about this skeleton. Most friends were aware I did not enjoy cooking but most people (including me) did not understand why. I think
this was the first skeleton I met.

Driving

Driving has been quite troubling for close to twenty years. During the 1980's
I worked as a case manager for several social service agencies. One responsibility was car travel throughout the state of Illinois. On average, I drove approximately 20,000 miles per year visiting schools, hospitals, social service
agencies, state government meetings, and long term care facilities. I entered
Graduate School at the University of Texas in Austin the fall of 1989. During
the first part of the 1990's I spent an enormous time on the highway—
traveling from Dallas to Austin, San Antonio, and Corpus Christi. I experienced my "feelings" while driving—so much so that I made mistakes.

I was driving home from Austin when I felt the "feeling." I was on highway 35 where the split took place—I couldn't decide and ended up in Forth Worth. God I was scared—what is this (spring 1991 personal journal)?

Because of the "feelings" I was consistently nervous about driving. I always preferred to drive alone. If I had a seizure while driving no one else would notice. If I was with a licensed driver at anytime that person would drive. Friends visiting me from other towns and states would drive my car while in town. I never connected this fear to consistent seizures. Most states enforce driving barriers for epileptics. Those experiencing a grand mal seizure are not to drive within six months. However, most states have not placed driving restrictions on those experiencing partial seizures. I did not own the severity of my seizures until 1998.

It has been too long since I have written—too much has happened. I had a serious car accident on January 23—because of a [partial] seizure. I was driving home from work and the seizure happened—I don't remember the accident— maybe images vaguely—I remember the seizure beginning and I could tell it was going to be serious. I never turned on Lake Dam—I stayed on Avent Ferry and ran off the road—drove over a big ditch—I don't even know how—and hit a tree. I wasn't seriously injured but had two months of pain in my chest. I don't drive anymore—not safe. I'm glad I didn't get hurt worse or hurt someone else. But my independence over—I am depending on others to get me around (March 21, 1998 personal journal).

I surrendered my license at this time. I knew it was not safe for me or others if I continued driving. I was able to legally drive in all fifty states a year after my last seizure in the hospital. However, it took me two years of seizure-free time before I was willing to purchase a car. The fear of the car accident was still strong.

Crossing Streets/Using Stairs

Walking has been very therapeutic for me over the years. It is great physical exercise and it has helped burn stress. The amount of miles I have walked has increased dramatically since the first diagnosed seizure in 1991. As much as I loved to walk I now am meeting one of the fear skeletons in the closet: using stairs and crossing streets.

I have had many seizures while using stairs and crossing streets. I always told myself what I should do if I happened to experience a seizure. However, I could not retrieve these instructions while seizing. According to friends and my own memories, I would always continue to move during a seizure. I would continue to cross a street and finish going up or down a flight of stairs.

I was usually quite lucky. Although I have tripped on the stairs many times I never fell down a flight. I was able to grasp the banister so tightly while climbing. A friend tells me I always clenched whatever was in my hands—so much so that I rarely spilled drinks during a seizure.

> I knew you were seizing. I tried to take your coffee out of your hands but your fist was so tightly wrapped around the mug—you didn't even spill any (conversation with Linda Tarkowski, Fall 1999).

Several times I would perform the act a few times. While experiencing a "bad" seizure I would go up and down the same flight of stairs a few times. If friends or colleagues noticed this I would be quite embarrassed. I was able to mumble that I forgot something and thus I need to go up or down the stairs once again.

Now, crossing streets was a different matter. This skeleton never trusted "walk" lights. Many times I crossed the street twice while seizing. During the seizure I couldn't understand the difference between green "walk" and red "walk." Thus, I would just cross the street again during the seizure. I vaguely remember a few car horns as I was crossing the street. This indicated to me that I was crossing the street against the "walk" light. I was never hit by a car or caused an accident at an intersection. I was very lucky.

Taking a Bath/Swimming Alone

I have always loved water. So much so that friends have called me the "water baby." In 1991 (as a result of my first diagnosed grand mal seizures) I became afraid of swimming alone or taking a bath. From 1991 to 1994 I lived in a condominium in Dallas, Texas with several pools and outdoor hot tubs. I always made sure there were other adults around when I entered a pool or hot tub. Still, I was never completely relaxed. I didn't anticipate a grand mal seizure (because of medications) but I still experienced at least thirty complex partial seizures per month. It was hard to relax in a bathtub or pool. I became nervous entering the water beginning in 1991 and this did not end until after surgery.

Deadlines

Our life is directed by "deadlines." Most of my friends, acquaintances, and co-workers test deadlines—i.e. turning in papers, projects, bills, reports—etc. on the last day. I have never tested deadlines and have quite a history of meeting required deadlines. In fact, I have been thanked by so many people over the years for turning required material in early—well before deadlines. This has been a consistent pattern for over twenty-five years. Even a few years ago I could not have totally explained why but I now can. Because I experienced up to ninety seizures per month, because I never knew when they would occur, and because I could never anticipate the severity I never tested deadlines. If I waited until the last moment to turn in a project and I then experienced a seizure the project may be delinquent. If this occurred more than once, it could call into question my professional capabilities.

This ambition spread throughout my life. As a student I read books, finished papers, projects, and studied and completed exams well before the due date. I arrived at airports to board a plane or pick up travelers well before departure or arrival times. I arrived in class early as a student or faculty member. I graded exams and turned in final grades early. I woke up early each morning, showered, dressed, and ate well before I would need to leave for jobs. I arrived early at every job I have held for twenty-five years. I arrived at all scheduled meetings early. I ordered books early for every class I ever taught. I wrote tests early for every class I taught and turned them into the copy center before most other faculty members.

I never followed deadlines imposed by others: I wrote my own deadlines constructed on a seizure-oriented clock. Thus, for most of my life I was early. My motto was: hurry up to wait. This seemed better than pressing imposed deadlines. If I followed other's deadlines I may have been late with projects as a result of consistent seizures.

Emotions

My emotions have been bottled-up for twenty-five years. I didn't experience reality much. Mostly, all I felt was seizures—the "feeling." Emotions were alive but buried deep in the closet. I rarely cried. Regardless of the personal loss I had a "flat" response. I smiled and laughed a great deal but rarely expressed deep emotions inside. I rarely expressed anger. For a long time I felt I did not understand anger. I now know this was not true. I was angry at the seizures but afraid to express this emotion. Denial was accepting. I denied I would continue seizing. I denied I was angry at this condition. Now it is time to acknowledge this anger and forgive the brain. My mother has felt guilty regarding this seizure condition. I never blamed her or the medical profession—I always blamed my brain—it was weak, very weak. But I could never identify or express that anger. I never felt "excited" about the future—never anticipated happiness. Somewhere inside I knew the seizures would become more frequent and intense. I had fun in life but never knew this until the event was over.

So it is time to notice that skeleton. I have failed to express and notice emotions. I was rarely angry, sad, happy, or excited. Basically, I was "flat" and afraid. That "emotions" skeleton hid in the corners of the closet—not wanting to be noticed by the other skeletons.

Difficulty Sleeping

I always knew I was a light sleeper. I would wake up several times each night. I always thought this was just a part of my character. I guess it was strongly correlated with my history of seizures. For the past twenty-five years I rarely experienced REM (rapid eye movement) or deep sleep. Thus, I did not experience dreams as often as other people. Apparently my brain was never totally relaxed. I never told many people about this condition. I never fully understood it. I have always felt tired most of the day but I rarely slept peacefully. According to my current neurologist (Kevan VanLandingham) my brain was always "popping." My brain was never "relaxed." I went to bed earlier (10:00 p.m.) and woke up later than others (8:00 a.m.). Thus, I tried to give my brain ten hours of sleep each night. Many times I took naps in the afternoon to reinforce brain rest and strength. However, I never felt "refreshed." I always felt I was carrying weights on my shoulders. I was always tired. I never told others about this condition—I was not truthful to myself. I felt each night would reinforce the brain. This was a tired skeleton that tried to get out of the closet every day. But that poor skeleton constantly needed to lean up against the wall of the closet to gain strength to survive.

Side Effects of Medications

Nausea

In the spring of 1998 seizure intensity increased significantly. I also experienced another Grand Mal seizure. As a result of this, I pursued treatment from another neurologist. At this time it was suggested I begin an additional medication: Depakote. I began taking this medication in the early summer of 1998. Although seizures did decrease in frequency, I continued to experience about one a day and intensity remained high. The side effects of Depakote were challenging. I imagine some patients could tolerate this medication but I was quite sensitive. I experienced a new side effect: nausea. Nausea was constant but I struggled the most at night. For the first six months I was very sick every night. Nausea would begin about 8:00 p.m. and last until about midnight. I would spend a few hours of every evening on the floor of my bathroom. I needed to take the medications and developed a schedule where I would be sure they were absorbed before nausea increased. I was continually nauseous for three years (summer 2001 I was able to retire the medication) and avoided a variety of foods I once adored. I lost my attraction to Italian foods, sauces, oils, salad dressings, meats in general, and any food with a strong taste. I became attracted to very bland foods: bread, many cheeses, and peanut butter. I was never hungry and meals were a challenge. I began counting calories to ensure an appropriate diet.

I constantly worked at constructing a daily schedule to avoid the "tough" hours. Teaching morning and evening classes were a risk and I needed to negotiate semester schedules on a regular basis. I realize (after talking to medical support staff) that although I was sensitive to Depakote, the increase in seizure intensity contributed to nausea. My brain never relaxed and was constantly out of balance.

Double Vision

Double vision is a side effect of a medication I was taking: Tegretol. Early morning was the most difficult time. Double vision weakens visual capabilities. I tripped a great deal. I wouldn't see small holes in sidewalks and misjudged curbs. Thus, I tripped several times each day walking to and from campus. I tripped going up and down stairs by misjudging distance. I learned to grasp banisters and guard rails.

This "side effect" skeleton has tried to get out of the closet so many times. However, many times this poor skeleton bumped into walls or was lying on the floor with severe nausea.

ACCEPTING THE SKELETONS

It is now time to meet and accept the skeletons. I have seen them many times but constantly pushed them into the closet. The lights in the closet are now on and I have left the door open. I can own and accept physical impairments. I have made an enormous amount of growth. I have not experienced a seizure since August of 2001 and my memory is strong. I have few fears, cope with deadlines, enjoy a range of emotions, sleep peacefully, and endure lighter side effects of medications. Indeed these are fantastic gains since surgery. The most important gain, however, is accepting the skeletons. For the rest of my life I will accept my faults and weaknesses. I may experience another seizure, I may experience memory impairments (due to aging), I will feel a fear or two in life, embrace new emotions, experience side-effects of other medications, and perhaps have difficulty sleeping a night or two. However, I will never close that closet door again. I will accept my skeletons—not imprison them.

NOTES

1. A "skeleton in the closet" refers to unpleasant secrets, old scandals (Prairie House Books 1995–2002).

2. Complex partial seizures involve impairment or loss of consciousness. Alteration of consciousness refers to lack of understanding. An individual is able to move about in a relatively normal manner but is, at the same time, suddenly lacking full understanding. Most complex partial seizures last for 1 to 3 minutes. Sometimes complicated behaviors occur during a complex partial seizure. These often involve partial undressing, urination, or other socially embarrassing behavior (Leppik 2000).

Chapter Six

Releasing An Imprisoned Spirit
Fall of 2001

Life is Given, Living is Something to Achieve

The Sixth Step of Recovery for Adult Children of Alcoholics
(www.geocities.com/howitworks2001/)
We give to God [higher power] as we know him, all former pain, hurt and mistakes, resentments and bitterness, anger and guilt. We trust that we can let go of the hurt.

I am not sure who I am anymore. A new part of me is alive—conceived in fear and born out of loneliness—a new part that functions on the streets of Raleigh, North Carolina. It is she that I am now just getting to know—beginning to notice—learning to accept. I have feelings and emotions I did not know I was capable of experiencing.

REVISITING SPIRITUALITY

I would like to reiterate my description of Spirituality. Spirit is hope, peace, energy, love, conviction, and pursuit of truth through a "higher power." I do not mean religious in any form. My higher power is my future—a stronger, healthier, happier, and peaceful Karen Glumm. I would like to describe the accomplishments of this "spirit" once released from "epileptic prison." First, I will describe the physical losses and gains.

PHYSICAL LOSSES AND GAINS

Losses

On August 15, 2001 I experienced invasive neurological surgery—a tangerine size chunk of brain were the seizures was housed were removed. As a result of this surgery I expected a series of physical losses. I can clearly describe these new limitations.

Eyesight

It seems that some of my eye muscles have changed since neurosurgery. I am aware that aging leads to near-sighted weakness. However, as a result of surgery I believe my eyes aged about fifteen years. Literally overnight I experienced weakness in my eyes—particularly viewing anything close-up. I have trouble reading (especially small type) and I am glad I have never been involved in sewing. I need bright lights while reading and I am constantly adjusting books and papers. However, this seems to be a small price.

Fine Motor Skills

I have always had weak fine motor skills. However, they have declined since neurosurgery. Although weak, I could easily write and read my own handwriting. Until now. Since surgery I have difficulty writing (weaker fine motor muscles) and I have trouble reading my handwriting. I have had to slow down while writing and type notes/ideas as soon as possible. I now have difficulty picking up small items such as paperclips, toothpicks, coins, and pens/pencils. I have trouble cutting meat and using scissors. Tasks utilizing fine motor skills tend to take a great deal more time now and I have to be much more careful than I did in the past. However, this has been a small price.

Phantom Pain

Every now and then I experience phantom pains—particularly in my hands. Suddenly I may feel a strange sharp pain in the fingertips of one of my hands—usually left hand. There is no known cause of this pain—I have had no known injury. The pain lasts for just a few minutes and then dissipates quickly. The frequency has decreased significantly but I still experience phantom pain every week or two. Prior to surgery I experienced a severe headache a few times every week as a result of serious complex partial seizures. I think this new pain, although strange, is much less painful than thirty to ninety seizures per month and consistent headaches.

Tingling

After surgery I began to feel "tingling" in both hands and feet on a consistent basis. The more I talked and walked the stronger the tingling. During the past few years this has decreased significantly but I still feel a consistent tingling in all my fingertips. The more physically or mentally active I am the greater the tingling and the more likely it will spread to all toes. It seems pretty strange but I recognize the "tingling" as my new "feeling"—a new feeling I embrace.

Headaches

I have headaches on a fairly consistent basis. If I ever concentrate on my head I will feel low grade pain in the left side. This is minor pain that I rate a one or a two on a ten point scale (ten is high). I figure having brain surgery in my forties would indicate lasting physical discomfort. When I physically exercise pain will gradually increase. When intensely reading or writing I will feel greater pain. However, this pain, on my personal scale is minor. I rarely take medications for pain. If I feel a stronger headache I reach for over-the-counter medications. This pain is very minor when considering the headaches I experienced while seizing thirty to ninety times per month.

Dent

As a result of surgery I now have a "dent" in the left side of my head—not far to the left of my left eye. This dent has about a one-inch circumference and is a few centimeters deep. This area is a bit sensitive to touch. Dr. Kevan VanLandingham (neurologist) suggested plastic surgery to "pad" this area. I did not even consider plastic surgery. I think I needed the "dent" as a souvenir —this crater seems to remind me of the twenty-five years of seizures. I know where the seizures lived and I touch that spot everyday—glad to know that that piece of brain is gone forever.

These losses are very minor when compared to physical accomplishments.

Gains

I hoped for a reduction in seizures but I never anticipated the physical gains I have experienced. This has been quite a surprise and celebration.

Energy

As noted, I experienced 30–90 seizures for over twenty-five years. If possible to conceptualize, there is something a bit worse than the seizure patterns themselves. My brain was never relaxed. I can now feel the difference. No matter how much sleep I received I was always tired. As a result of this I had little energy. Walking, reading, and talking became a chore. Now I see the dramatic difference. I have an incredible amount of energy. I wake up ready to begin a schedule. In the past I needed two hours every morning before I could ask the brain to work. Now the brain works before the body is fully awake. During the seizure lifestyle, all I did during the early morning hours was shower, drink coffee, and have breakfast. I needed the brain to just "be"—I could never "think." That is over—so much so that I need blank pages and pens everywhere to note ideas and plans I have for the day, week, or year. My brain begins to work before 7:00 a.m. and does not quit until well after midnight. These hours are set by the body—not the brain. This is a new experience for me. I have an "active" brain and I embrace the energy—a quality I am just now beginning to notice and celebrate.

Sleep

I have read a great deal about the value of "deep" REM (rapid eye movement) sleep. This is the healthiest sleep: allowing the body and mind to rest and revitalize. What I did not realize until now is that I have not experienced this sleep pattern much during the past twenty-five years. I now know because I experience deep, pleasant sleep every night. In the past I woke up about ten times per night. Apparently, my brain was never "relaxed." Even while not seizing my brain was disturbed. So much so that as noted I was always tired but rarely experienced the REM deep sleep. I went to bed every night about 10:00 p.m. and woke up at 8:00 a.m. Still, my brain was always tired. I did not anticipate this physical "gain." I had no idea my brain was worn out twenty-four hours a day. Finally, my brain is at peace and I enjoy deep sleep.

Gross Motor

My gross motor capabilities have increased significantly since my last seizure. Before surgery I tripped while walking and stumbled on staircases. When turning corners in buildings I would bump into the walls (misjudge space) and constantly bruised my hips, shoulders, hands, and feet. I many times bumped my head by misjudging space. This rarely happens at this time. I no longer need to grasp banisters so tightly and I am much more confident and relaxed while walking the streets. My competence in spatial decisions has grown significantly. As much as I tried to blame my incompetence on medications, I now realize that the side-effects were not the main cause. I am still on medications and I feel stable while walking, climbing stairs, turning corners, and bending under furniture/tables. I think my seizure-oriented brain was out of focus and had difficulty predicting spatial areas.

Memory

One of my strongest physical gains is my memory. As seizures increased in frequency and intensity I experienced greater problems with memory. When I agreed to endure surgery to reduce seizures I did not ask for a stronger memory—I just asked for my memory to no longer deteriorate. One of the many pleasant gifts I received from the surgery is receiving the strongest memory I have had for twenty-five years. I no longer need to keep as many notes as I did in the past. I still have a pattern to note appointments and accomplishments but I remember events on a regular basis. I remember names, addresses, and phone numbers. The greatest gift, however, is old memories returning. I remember experiences from childhood, teenage years, young adulthood, and yesterday. Many people may not realize what a gift this new memory is to me. Over the past twenty years I have felt my memory slipping. The four years prior to surgery significantly impacted my memory bank. Now, each day, I remember past experiences (I even celebrate the not-so-pleasant memories). Finally, all 1,000 pieces of my spirit are once again falling into place. I am rejuvenated—I spend a great deal of time pulling old memories and ideas out of the archives. Although dusty, those pieces of the spirit are alive and doing well inside this new soul. On a regular basis I play mind "games" to constantly exercise my brain. I realize I will always have some trouble with memory but I have learned to reduce pressure. I experience every moment and its connection to the past and future. At this time I celebrate my new "hard drive." I guess this hard drive is a bit smaller than the old one but it has thousands of old files and an incredible amount of available storage space.

Alert

I have recently discovered that I am so much more alert than ever before in my life. I can respond to events and make immediate decisions when necessary. During the ten years before surgery I learned to allow increasing amounts of time making serious decisions. I seemed to move "slower" than the rest of the universe. My brain was in slow motion and I learned how to manage this speed. Well, my mental engine can now move faster than twenty miles per hour. In fact, I think for the first time in my life my brain moves faster than the rest of my body. Perhaps I realize the frustration a two year old child experiences.

White Clouds Replace Dark Clouds

Dark Clouds moved into my mental sky during the past ten years. Five years prior to surgery these clouds were crowding my sky. These were heavy clouds which minimized natural light and suggested heavy storms. Still today my mind has some clouds. However, now these are white clouds. Many days my sky has no clouds at all. Every few days I will see some white clouds. Maybe briefly one of the white clouds will pass over the sun and cause brief shade. However, just wait a few moments and the sun will return. I have been experiencing a beautiful sky. I never recognized the beauty of the sky—my dark clouds limited vision and understanding of the mental sky.

Sense of Gravity

Gradually, over the years, my sense of gravity declined significantly (as a result of the increase in medications and seizure severity). Until now I could not fully recognize the difference. During the ten years prior to surgery, I consistently felt dizzy and nauseous. I never felt grounded. I have blamed this on medications (which may have contributed to nausea) but I can now relate this discomfort to the epileptic brain. I was never grounded and always felt dizzy. I am still talking anti-seizure medications and I, for the first time in well over ten years, feel a sense of gravity.

RELEASING IMPRISONED SPIRIT

Ideas, aspirations, hope, emotions, and innovations of the spirit have been imprisoned by the epileptic. Now it is time to release the spirit—encourage recognition and growth of the soul.

Critical Moment

Following Gamson (1992) I acknowledge that "critical moments" can make discourse on an issue visible as they stimulate commentary. To gather the energy and courage to release the imprisoned spirit I needed the critical moment. This moment occurred during the early stage of recovery. I can't remember the exact day but it was in October of 2001—I rewrote life. I no longer calculated a day based on how many seizures I experienced, the severity of the seizures, the social implications of seizures, and the side-effects of medications. Finally, I woke up asking myself not when I would seize but what I would experience. I began to relearn life—seizures no longer controlled my soul. My mind was free—free to experience life fully and realistically.

Decrease of Rituals

In October of 2001 I was ready to decrease daily rituals. During my seizure lifestyle most of my time was spent fearing seizures, trying to reduce seizures, and treating seizures. All my time was constructed by a seizure-oriented clock. I was ready to decrease my ritualistic behavior. I learned how to let my mind wander the universe. I never set a schedule. I let my brain decide when to wake up. I ate what I wanted when I actually felt hungry. I began traveling around town whenever I wanted. I called friends and family members when I wanted—I no longer had an internal seizure-clock. For ten years prior to surgery I followed a schedule set in advance—changed only by a seizure. Now, I write a schedule as I live—allowing the spirit to delete any event and add another.

New Interests

I now have new goals and ambitions. I have always been a writer. I have written and published several articles and I am conducting other social research. As much as I have enjoyed writing, mental exercises became "hard work" during the past ten years. As a result of increased seizure activity my mind was weakening. I was losing depth in constructing sentences, building paragraphs, and transcribing life through words. Now, as a result of the removal of my seizure focal point, writing is considerably easier. My mental "thesaurus" is deeper than it has been for my entire life. In fact, writing is my interaction with the universe. This was my ambition when I was young. I remember traveling across the country several times trying to record my experiences. My literate "hard drive" is once again alive each minute of the day. Rather than constantly "reacting" in life I am now interacting with life. I visit malls, ride city buses, sit in coffee shops, and walk the streets to meet and interact with life. Sleep is now a requirement not a choice. Living is now a choice not a requirement.

Love of Music

When young I loved music. I think music was always my expression of life. On a very slow pace the fifteen years prior to surgery I lost this passion. I rarely listened to music. Even at Christmas I turned volume low. I think the brain was "too busy" for music—especially as the focal point spread. My love of music is returning. Every night I spend a few hours with the headphones on—listening to a range of musicians. While writing, thinking, relaxing, and living I want music in the background. I express and celebrate life with music. This spirit has returned and enjoys time.

Facing Death

I now enjoy every moment of life. I think I began to greatly appreciate life when I learned I had been so close to death the first few weeks after neurosurgery. The first ten days after surgery I slipped into a coma twice. From what I understand, many friends and medical support staff felt I might die as a result of complications during this stage of recovery. Well, I didn't. My body continued to fight—reaching for and eventually grabbing life. I am an agnostic—doubting the presence of the Christian God. Fearing death is a possible side-effect to being an agnostic. The greatest benefit to Christianity is the acceptance of "after-life." I am not criticizing Christianity. However, I doubt after-life. As a result of this belief I have feared death for twenty-five years.

However, I almost died twice shortly after brain surgery. I remember slipping away twice and I remember returning. As a result of this life threatening condition I no longer fear death. When death has to arrive I'll slip away once again. In the meantime, I will enjoy life. I believe this experience taught me how to celebrate life—every moment.

Emotional Growth

I never anticipated such emotional growth. For the first time in my life I am "centered." I am now experiencing a complete range of emotions. More importantly, I accept this range. Emotions are part of a soul. I'm sure I make mistakes: emotional responses are never perfect. However, I accept my emotional responses and I will apologize if necessary. I notice and accept my weaknesses. I enjoy the responses to life. Most importantly, I celebrate my ability to "feel" and "express" life.

Releasing the Skeletons

I now know that my brain was not weak but quite strong. So strong that it endured twenty-five years of seizures. Indeed this brain "bounced back" after surgery. It is time to release the skeletons from the closet. Rather than feel fear or embarrassment regarding my deficiencies it is time to celebrate. Even while having so many seizures, coping with memory losses and drug side-effects, and experiencing fears and tight emotions for twenty-five years I pressed on. I constantly tested my limitations and accomplished a great deal. My weaknesses are a part of my history and personality.

Mourning

I was discharged from Duke Hospital on August 29, 2001. I still had a considerable period of recovery—more than I anticipated. I learned to talk, walk, and think again. For the first time in my life I cried every day. At the time I believed I was learning how to express emotions. As a child of an alcoholic with seizures I "bottled" my emotions for many years and I was beginning to express pain, suffering, fear, and happiness. I believe most people use tears to express these emotions—I never had. In the fall of 2001 I learned to express and accept emotions: I could now cry in front of others.

As much as I believe this was true during the fall of 2001, I had more to accept. In early 2002 I realized the tears continued. After serious soul searching I realized I was mourning. I experienced seizures for over twenty-five years. Experiencing, tolerating, and coping with seizures was a time consuming lifestyle—so much so that I missed a great deal of living. So beginning spring of 2002 I began mourning the loss of expressing my true spirit for over twenty-five years. I am extremely happy at the age of 47—enjoying life, celebrating who I am, and anticipating an exciting future. However, I can't help but mourn the losses during the twenty-five years experiencing chronic seizures. As glad as I am to meet and live with this Karen Glumm, I wish I had met her during my late teens. I think an endless supply of tears expresses these losses.

CELEBRATING LIFE

I believe I am experiencing some type of "midlife crisis." This concept was constructed to describe a period of emotional turmoil in middle age. The turmoil especially indicates a strong desire for change (Merriam-Webster 2003). At this time in my life I am experiencing a strong desire for emotional change.

I never knew what "celebrating" life meant. For twenty-five years I lived day-by-day—coping with seizures, tolerating side-effects of medications, accomplishing projects before, during, and after seizures, and recovering from seizures.

In the past three years I have learned how to celebrate life. I enjoy every moment of the day. I don't care when or what I eat, where I am, what time of day it is, who I am with, or what my schedule requires. I enjoy time.

Every day, every hour, every minute, and every second is a celebration of life. I can now understand what most people have seen, heard, smelled, enjoyed, and hated for all their lives. This is so new to the seizure-free mind. It is now time to learn how to live in a seizure-free world.

If I stop walking for only a second I can hear the trees sprouting new leaves. If I look close enough I can see the grass growing before my eyes. So, please, for just a moment, let me utilize only my passport in the kingdom of the well.

Chapter Seven

Learning to Laugh
Mid-late Fall of 2001

"You grow up the day you have your first real laugh—at yourself"

(Unknown)

The Eleventh Step of Recovery for Adult Children of Alcoholics
(www.geocities.com/howitworks2001/)
We see through our own power and a Higher Power, awareness of our inner selves.
We do this through reading, listening, meditation, sharing, and other ways of centering.

LEARNING TO LAUGH AT MYSELF AS A
CHILD OF AN ALCOHOLIC

Seizure experiences are strange and many times embarrassing. Part of recovery is to understand and accept this condition. I am ready to share these experiences. I learned as a Social Services Worker that laughter inspires endorphins—natural body chemicals that help us cope with pain and stress. Coping with seizures for twenty-five years has, in a way, developed my personality. I like the person I am—seizure history and all. I learned to laugh at myself as a recovering child of an alcoholic fifteen years ago. Now it is time to laugh at my seizure lifestyle and all the mistakes I made. Please laugh with me.

SEIZURES (PARTIAL AND GRAND MAL) AROUND OTHERS

In 1991 I experienced my first Grand Mal and was placed on a drug regimen. Gradually, I added medications but seizure frequency and intensity increased.

As a result of this, I was losing control of myself while seizing. I could no longer hide the "feeling."

Grand Mal

I experienced my first Grand Mal (generalized) seizure on June 22, 1991. This seizure occurred in the middle of the night—well after I went to sleep. I don't remember the seizure. When I woke up I heard voices but I could not understand the language. I saw two men in my bedroom. This caused me to sit up and try to fight back if necessary. I recognized my roommate and at that time she rushed over to try to calm me down. She had a very serious look on her face and tried to explain that I had a seizure and the two men were paramedics. I could not understand a word she was saying. I could tell the two men were setting up a stretcher. I realized that the men were paramedics. I could barely move and did not understand language so figured they were there for me but I had no idea why. For several minutes I heard the paramedics and Linda talking but I could not understand a word. Finally, I could interpret language. One of the paramedics turned to Linda and said "why don't you help her put a shirt on?" Finally, on my way to the hospital in the ambulance I realized Linda was trying to tell me I had a grand mal seizure.

Medical intervention was difficult and tiring that night. Medical staff continued to ask questions to determine the cause of the seizure. Linda was filling out papers so I was alone with staff. I was asked how long it took for me to recover from the seizure. I didn't know. She then asked the first words I could understand. I used to be a social service worker and I understood personal records. This woman didn't care what she wrote down as long as she filled in the blank. I certainly did not want those first words I understood to become a part of my permanent file. My mind was blurry and working slow but I worked hard to come with other words that were true and I could always recall if asked. She asked me a few times and I told her "I'm working on it." Finally, I looked at her and said "the first words I understood was my roommate telling me I experienced a seizure." This seemed to satisfy the medical staff and she wrote that down in the empty blank. Of course, I still remember those were "the first words" I remember.

Partial Seizures

I have had hundreds of partial seizures around others for the past twenty years. During the ten years prior to surgery the intensity and frequency of the seizures increased and thus my behavior during seizures was increasingly odd and noticeable. The most common result of complex seizures was the difficulty to speak or understand language. Many times I could not speak or understand what others were saying during a partial seizure. This could last only a few seconds or up to an hour (during a very tough partial seizure). I knew I was having a seizure but I didn't know how to tell others. After years of training as a social service worker I was able to read body language. I could tell that others around me knew I was having a seizure and they were concerned. I tried to leave a room full of people and seek a private space. People always followed me asking questions. I'm sure they were concerned but there was no way I could communicate. Over time I began to create patterned responses: "I'll be okay soon, just leave me alone;" "tell the class I can return soon, just leave me alone;" or "this is a bad one so please leave me alone." Perhaps I should have created these as signs back in 1994.

As seizures increased in intensity in 1998 I experienced new behavior. The new response was strange gestures and swallowing. Linda Tarkowski remembers times I would raise my left arm like I was ready to dribble a basketball. I would hold this arm out for several minutes. When out in public Linda would try to lower this arm. Apparently I blocked traffic in several restaurants. I'm sure this "strange" behavior attracted attention as I tried to dribble a basketball while sitting in a restaurant.

During this same time period I remember "swallowing" during bad seizures. I would feel the seizure increase in intensity and I think I was trying to swallow the seizure. I can imagine what others thought while I was swallowing, getting ready to dribble a non-existent basketball, and couldn't understand a word anyone else said.

Car Accident

As a result of a severe partial seizure I experienced a car accident in the spring of 1998. It is now time to celebrate the fact that I recovered from this accident and did not hurt anyone else. I remember the seizure starting but I lost consciousness quite quickly. When I regained consciousness a young man was knocking on my door asking if I was ok. I felt a bit disoriented but I felt fine. Then I looked up and noticed there was a huge crack in my windshield. My car was up against a large tree. Did the city plant trees in the middle of the road? The young man asked if I was able to leave the car. Actually, I felt fine so I got out. I was able to notice that the car was ruined. I was quite lucky to have survived that accident (and not hurt anybody else). When the police officer arrived he seemed a little surprised to see the car ruined and me walking fine. The officer asked me to "walk around." I figured he was giving me a field sobriety test. However, I was cold stone sober and still ran into that tree. The cop seemed convinced I was a traditional "woman driver" and thus

I slid off a slippery road into a tree. I was willing to accept this stereotype and thus did not have to describe the seizure. I stopped driving after this accident. I have visited the tree and found a piece of my car and I have this as a souvenir. I can legally drive in all fifty states and have a car. I try to stay away from trees.

ADJUSTING TO MEDICATIONS

For ten years (1991–2001) I was on a tight medication regimen. Over time, dosage was increased and new medications added. During these ten years I tried four different medications and continued to experience 30–90 seizures every month. Each medication had a series of side effects. One of my major accomplishments as a victim of epilepsy was "insight." I knew I was frequently seizing even while taking a series of medications. So as horrid as the side effects were, I knew I needed to continue to take medications on a regular basis. It is time to laugh at these patterns and side effects.

Possible Facial Hair/Hair Loss/Possible Facial Hair

My history of anti-seizure medications has been very interesting regarding facial hair and hair loss. These two medications are Depakote and Dilantin.

Dilantin was the first anti-seizure medication prescribed in the summer of 1991. This is one of the oldest medications (and most reliable) for epileptics. One of the strongest side-effects of Dilantin is an increase in facial hair. After being on this medication only three months I began to notice a slight increase in facial hair. I dropped this medication in the spring of 1992 (Tegretol was prescribed for partial seizures) and I quickly lost that moustache. I was glad that hair left my body. However, I didn't realize what would happen with Depakote.

Men tend to be the most vulnerable to "receding hairlines" or baldness. My father and one of my brothers consistently lost hair. I was quite proud to be a female with a full head of hair. Until Depakote. One of the many side-effects of Depakote is impact on hair roots. During the summer of 1998 I started losing hair. From the summer of 1998 until the summer of 2001 I had a great deal in common with my brothers. My bathtub drain began clogging because of hair. My combs and brushes were full of hair. My bathroom floor was littered with hair. During this three year period my hair was thinning.

After neurosurgery I was no longer prescribed Depakote. On my head I can see the difference. My hair feels thicker. I can see waves and character in my hair for the first time in several years. My hairbrushes and combs feel they have less work to do. My bathtub drains easily. Finally, I don't have to vacuum my bathroom floor as often. I once again feel free from my family's "receding" hairline. In fact, I had a new battle. I am still taking anti-seizure medications. Dilantin was once again prescribed after surgery. While on this medication I checked my face every day looking for a mustache. I began to see a few hairs. All of my friends say they did not see any facial hairs. I did see a moustache and this continued for the first three years after surgery. Finally, after four years seizure-free, dilantin was removed from my regimen. The mustache was removed and I celebrated recovery once again.

Diplopia

In the spring of 1992 I was encouraged to try a new medication: Tegretol. Tegretol was noted as the best performing drug for partial seizures. I took this drug for nine years: Spring of 1992 to Summer of 2001. Looking back over the past nine years I can say this drug was not as successful as I hoped. I did tolerate the side effects but they were troubling. The most difficult and common side effect was diplopia—double vision. This was kinda like living in a Double Mint Gum commercial. Approximately an hour after taking the medication I would experience double vision. I took the medication right after waking up and late in the evening. Mornings were the most difficult. Hot showers and physical exercise stimulated the double vision. So I woke up, took the medication, showered, and walked to campus. By the time I reached the halfway point the double vision kicked in. I frequently stumbled because I could not see the cracks on the sidewalk and failed to see holes in the street. I tripped going up and down stairs because I misjudged the distance between steps. I learned to grasp banisters to ensure stability.

My first class of the day was Research Methods and Statistics. I would still have double vision many times during this class. While working out problems on the board in front of the class I would close one eye to be sure I didn't make mistakes with statistical formulas. Students seemed confused and a bit jealous that I could do the math with "one eye closed." This double vision tapered off late in the morning. I have not taken Tegretol since my brain surgery. I can really "see the difference." I only see one of everything.

I did not realize until now all the side effects of Tegretol. Now I see details. I can easily cross streets, I don't stumble, and I can go up and down stairs without grasping banisters. I think I always walked slow—fearing that the epileptic inside of me would fall. Now I walk faster—in fact—I'm running.

Nausea

As mentioned in chapter 5, my seizure intensity increased in the spring of 1998. At this time I began taking a new medication: Depakote. I experienced a new side effect: nausea. For the first three months on Depakote I was physically ill every night. I learned to grade homework/tests and write lectures at certain times of the day. Of course toward the end of the semester I was very busy so I had to grade between pukes. I learned how to balance these two events well. At this time my neurologist (and friends) encouraged me to smoke marijuana. This was a major flashback to undergraduate days in the 1970's. A friend of mine was able to find marijuana and I once again was going to smoke a joint. I bought a "one hitter" pipe and this made smoking marijuana easier. The marijuana was able to relax my brain and nausea would dissipate. This experience lasted a few months.

Eventually I was somewhat balanced but I continued to experience nausea early in the morning and the evening. I usually walked to school at 9:30 a.m. every morning and home between 3:00–5:00 p.m. I had to pass a Kentucky Fried Chicken Fast Foods restaurant twice a day. Can you imagine the impact on my nausea? For several blocks twice a day I endured the scent and battled nausea. Several times a day I would go to the student union center. The main restaurant in the Cate Center was Chick Filet. My nausea would once again kick in. A few of my colleagues brought Chick Filet lunch over to our office building each day. I will never eat fried chicken again. Students would offer to pick up lunch for me from the student union. Of course I said "no, I only eat yogurt for lunch." Actually I tried to avoid many foods but fried chicken was the worse.

Centrum Silver and Ensure

In the year of 1998 (in addition to 30–90 partial seizures per month) I experienced two grand mal seizures. As a result of these experiences I was prescribed a second medication (in addition to Tegretol): Depakote. Most drugs have side effects. In addition to nausea, Depakote depleted the body's supply of vitamins and minerals. As a result of this, my neurologist encouraged me to take a new multi-vitamin. At the age of forty I was encouraged to begin taking Centrum Silver—the multi-vitamin for the aged. I remember telling my 71 year old mother that I was taking this vitamin. Her response: "oh yes, I take that vitamin as well." Finally, my mother and I had something in common.

As a result of neurosurgery, I no longer take Depakote. However, my mother and I once again have something in common. As a result of neurosurgery and recovery I lost an enormous amount of weight. During rehabilitation I needed to increase body weight and protein intake (most of my friends were jealous because I was encouraged to gain weight). One intensive care nurse at Duke Hospital encouraged me to drink Ensure (concentrated liquid with protein and balanced vitamin supplements). In October of 2001 I told my mother I drank an Ensure every day to enhance protein and add calories. She seemed happy. She stated "I drink one every day." Once again we have something in common. So, with a can of Ensure in my hand I drink a toast to our common bonds.

GRADING BETWEEN SEIZURES

Every semester I taught four classes. Each class had at least three tests, a series of homework assignments, and one project. A great deal of my spare time was spent grading student's work. As my seizures increased in intensity and frequency I had to learn to grade between events. I learned to take notes on each student's test/homework papers. Students were surprised to receive such detail description of points. They did not realize I did that for my own "memory." On a fairly regular basis, I was grading and then experienced a seizure. I might have to put that paper aside for ten minutes or a few hours. After recovery, I was able to look at that paper and because of notes I wrote I was able to pick up where I left off. I learned how to adjust to my episodes. Now I can grade papers, read essays, and write papers without seizure episodes. I think I may have to come up with a new excuse for putting the papers aside for a period of time.

CO-WORKERS "WALKING" ME DOWN HALL

On September 23, 1999 I had a grand mal seizure on my campus. I was in the student computer lab across the hall from my office helping students with homework assignments. I don't remember the seizure starting but I do remember well the post-ictil stage. When I "came" to I could hear the voices of a group of people around me. I couldn't understand the words but I could tell by eye contact that I was the subject. They all looked very concerned. I was lying on the floor trying to get up—I wanted out of that room. I wanted to be alone (without anyone talking about me until I could understand the language). Slowly, after a seizure, capabilities begin to come back. First, I could breath, then hear (although I could not interpret the speech), then eyesight, and next was physical strength (walking). The last to return for me was language interpretation. I couldn't speak or understand language. I knew I had a seizure.

The first thing I wanted to know was if I lost continence? Did I wet my pants? No, I could tell I was dry—good. This was an accomplishment. At this time I wanted to get up and walk across the hall to my office—to be alone. I was a bit unstable—muscles are very tired after a grand mal seizure. I was able to get up slowly. I did fall up against the table and a wall twice but I tried to walk. I wanted out of that room. Two people helped me up and helped me walk. I was not able to tell them where I wanted to go. I pointed out the door so they helped me leave the computer lab. However, instead of helping me walk across the hall to my office we turned right out the lab and continued walking down the hall. I couldn't understand what they were saying but I knew there were two choices at the end of the hall. To the right were several flights of stairs. To the left was the women's restroom. I did not have the physical capability to go down the stairs—I would have fallen a few flights. I did not have the need or the desire for the women's restroom. I couldn't speak, but like a two-year-old I tried to shake my head "no" but I was ignored. We kept walking. Eventually we turned left into the restroom. I shook my head no again. I was once again ignored. Into the stall we went. One of the women unbuckled my belt and began to pull down my pants. Finally, I was able to say "no—office." So, finally they walked me down the hall into my office and let me sit down in a comfortable chair to relax. I have never forgotten that experience and I still work on remembering the word "no." The two-year-old is still alive in my soul.

LOSS OF MEMORY

Over time, the increase in seizure intensity and frequency led to memory impairments. I realized I had picked the ideal profession. I was able to slide right into the stereotype of a college faculty member—the absent-minded professor. Students always reminded me of dates and details. I think they were proud to have a professor with memory impairments and always told me my mind must be so full of information that I couldn't remember tiny details. I was willing to have the "absent-minded professor" label stamped on my forehead. In fact, I would still like this imprint on my forehead.

TESTING

I entered Duke Hospital (Durham, NC) for testing on July 2, 2001. Dr. Kevan VanLandingham would conduct a series of tests to locate the seizure focal point. Once located, tests would be conducted to determine if removal of the focal point was possible. Over the past ten years I have been tested many times but the focal point was never determined. Upon intake I stopped taking all medications and was hooked up to a twenty-four hour EEG to locate the focal point. Dr. VanLandingham was interested in a series of seizures to ensure I had only one focal point.

Packing for Hospital—Denial

Prior to check-in, Kevan noted he would strip me of all medications to encourage seizures. He would also keep me awake for at least twenty-four hours. A "sleep-deprived" brain tends to have a much lower seizure threshold. I would be lying in bed for several days and awake for the first twenty-four hours. I figured I would have "extra" time on my hands during these days. I brought my laptop to continue working on my research project. I also brought books to continue reviewing past literature for my research topic. I also called the hospital in advance to ensure I could log onto the Internet. I wanted to check on the DOW and work on my research project. I was convinced I would work on the computer consistently. Obviously I was in a state of denial. I was going to have a series of seizures and thus I wouldn't have much energy to conduct research. However, I am a workaholic and thought this time was useful. I never opened the case with the computer—the laptop stayed in there for four days. In fact, after being awake eighteen hours I was so crabby that I wanted to hurl that laptop out my window. Hospital staff seemed amused when they saw all the stuff I brought. I couldn't think cognitively after being awake for twenty hours and I didn't give a damn about the DOW.

Teaching Hospital

Duke is a teaching hospital. Thus, every time a patient is visited by a physician a team of medical students tag along. I was visited many times by my neurologist and neurosurgeon. Thus, two teams of medical students visited me daily. I felt I was in a human zoo. All students wanted to read my chart, check incisions, and ask questions. I support teaching hospitals and I relied on this tolerance during my most trying times. I didn't want to see anybody during the twenty-four hours I stayed awake to inspire seizures. But I had to talk to all students. I didn't want to talk to anybody during surgery recovery because I was in pain and very uncomfortable. But I did allow all students to poke at my skull, offer IVs, change bandages, and ask questions that I could not answer. I had to plea for pain killers knowing they would have to ask the true doctor for approval.

Words To Remember

When I first started seeing Dr. VanLandingham he gave me three words to remember. This became the first question he asked me each time me met. During the entire testing period he asked me several times what were the three words. Prior to entering Duke Hospital I met with Dr. VanLandingham and he once again asked for the three words. I looked him in the eye and said "Kevan, after you remove a part of my brain I may only have three words in my vocabulary. Friends will ask what I wish for dinner and I will say 'tulip.' Others may notice I am upset and will ask if something is bothering me and I will say 'pear.' You may ask how I feel about my future and I will say 'courage.' That's it—I'll never have any additional words after I'm done here." However—Dr. VanLandingham has added three additional words to my vocabulary so I feel enriched. If a friend asks were I would like to live I can say "tree." If others ask why I appear angry I will be able to say "leader." If medical staff ask if I feel comfortable about my medical future I can say "honest."

Monitoring

I was closely monitored during the testing period. I was under twenty four hour surveillance by a camera. If I walked around the room the camera would follow me. Medical practitioners wanted to observe all physical movements during seizures several times to search for patterns. Thankfully the camera did not follow me into the restroom—I did have a bit or privacy. I did enter the restroom several times to avoid video tapes of all my behavior (i.e. change clothes, washing). I didn't want permanent records of all my actions.

I was on a cardiac monitor during this time period. I felt I had an eight pound baby strapped to my chest. As mentioned, I was hooked up to a twenty-four hour EEG. Thus, I could not leave the room. The cords were long enough that I could walk around that small room. I could use the restroom but no shower for several days. Medical staff took my vital signs every two hours: blood pressure, temperature, and pulse (even though I was hooked up to the cardiac monitor). The vein on my left arm was ready to accept medications if necessary. After I had a series of seizures I would be injected with valium to quiet the brain and reduce the chance of seizures. A friend of mine took several pictures of me during these days. I was looking forward to getting the valium.

Hoping For Seizures

My "wish list" was strange during this time period. For the first time in my life I "hoped" I would have a series of seizures. After being off medications for a few days I had my first severe complex partial seizure. I was so proud.

I hoped for more. Over the next few days I experienced three more severe complex partial seizures. I was so happy to offer pictures of my seizures. It was at this time that Dr. Kevan VanLandingham felt four seizures offered enough data to locate the seizure focal point. He wanted to give me Valium to quiet the focal point and put the brain to sleep. I was confused. I felt I could offer more seizures for the practitioners. Kevan convinced me that my seizure focal point was located and testing was complete. It was time "to sleep it off." So I accepted the Valium injection. Actually, the drug felt great and I enjoyed the long nap.

WADA

After testing, Kevan told me the seizure focal point was located in the left temporal lobe. At this time he was trying to gain information. He said "Karen I know you write with your right hand. Is it possible you were born left-handed but your mother taught you to write with your right hand?" I knew he was beating around the bush. So, I said "Kevan, you want to know if my left lobe is dominant. Why don't you try to figure it out. I'll give you information. Am I an artist? Why, yes, I can draw stick people. Do I like music? Why, yes, I am tone deaf but I love singing commercial songs. What were my favorite subjects? Math and Social Sciences. Eventually he was able to figure out I was left brain. Thus, the focal point was located in my dominant lobe. I needed a new test: WADA. This was a test developed by a female practitioner to determine the strength of each lobe independently. Twice I was injected with an anesthetic. My right lobe was tested first with the left lobe asleep. I wasn't able to speak, felt sedated, and I had double-vision. Thus I had some difficulty with the test. However, I was able to remember most of the pictures I was shown. Next, my left lobe was tested with my right asleep. I did not even feel the anesthetic. I did not have double-vision and I could speak just fine. I was able to answer all questions on the test. According to Kevan, my left lobe was dominant but my right lobe was strong enough. Thus, removal of part of my left lobe was now acceptable. My brain would remain strong enough.

SURGERY AND POST-SURGERY RECOVERY

Agnostic

I have always been an agnostic—doubting the presence of a God. I learned early that my neurosurgeon was a devout Christian. I certainly did not tell him I was an agnostic. A few hours before surgery Dr. Haglund came to my room to pray with me. I do not pray to a God. However, I did not need to press this issue. I held hands with Dr. Haglund and closed my eyes. He prayed he would do the best surgery possible. I certainly wanted that so silently looked to my higher power for him to do a good job.

Surgery

My memories of two weeks in Duke Hospital are cloudy and vague. However, I do have some that now inspire laughter.

I thought I would "sleep" through surgery. However, this did not happen. While performing surgery on my left brain lobe the surgeons woke me up several times to search for the location of "speech." I am right handed and thus speech was located in the left lobe. I think my friends wanted speech removed but my surgeon preferred to avoid removing this part of the brain. I was shown many pictures and asked many questions. I remember many times I was not able to answer any of the asked questions. I didn't understand why they were showing me stupid pictures in the middle of surgery. I was tired and wanted to sleep. Someone kept snapping his fingers to wake me up. Eventually, I was able to answer a few questions and finally I was able to sleep.

I spent several days in intensive care. I remember waking up in restraints a few times. According to Linda Tarkowski, I had tried to pull at bandages on my head several times so I was placed in restraints. When I woke up I would feel my face itching. This appears to be a side-effect of morphine. I could not reach my face because of the restraints. I also could not speak so I couldn't tell others my face was itchy. People wonder why I am always scratching my face now.

I remember feeling pain during this time as well. I couldn't talk and didn't know how to self-induce morphine. Linda was there and she could tell by my eyes and gestures that I was feeling pain so she would give me hits of morphine. I remember the pain going away. However, then the itching would start. I just tried to sleep as much as possible.

Apparently, I had difficulty breathing several days and thus was placed on a respirator. I remember waking up feeling the tube in my lungs. This was uncomfortable but my greatest fear was removal of this tube. I have watched so many medical shows on television and it has always seemed that the removal of this tube was uncomfortable and painful. As a child of an alcoholic I always "imagine" an event feeling worse than it will. This happened with the respirator. The removal of that tube did not feel uncomfortable. I think the hours of dreading this removal was far worse than the event itself.

The last few days of recovery in the hospital seemed great. My neurologist and neurosurgeon were discussing discharge. Before I could be discharged, however, I had to learn to use the restroom on my own. I had been on a catheter for almost two weeks. Every time I tried to enter the bathroom hospital staff would enter my room. Finally, Linda stood "watch" outside the room to enhance privacy. One of my favorite nurses, Owen, asked Linda what was going on. Linda was able to tell him I was having trouble learning how to use the restroom. At that time Owen came charging in the room telling me he could help. He gave me a few alcohol swabs and told me to smell them. Well, this worked. Finally, I learned how to use the restroom and I would be able to be discharged soon. I had graduated.

Post-Surgery Recovery

I was discharged from Duke Hospital August 29, 2001. I was still in recovery and many days were challenging.

I was taking nine different medications several times a day. One of those medications was sodium tablets. I had a shortage of sodium in my body. Because of this I could not drink many liquids during the day. I had to take nine different medications a few times per day and was not supposed to drink many fluids. Choking down those pills with a dry throat was very difficult. I had these dreams where I was in a desert and saw water. Unfortunately I woke up with a dry throat and a handful of pills to swallow. After about a week or two I was able to drink fluids once again and for the first time in many years I drank coke every day. Quite a celebration.

I am very happy that I only saw close friends and family members during the first couple months of recovery. Parts of my dominant left lobe were removed and my brain was swollen for several weeks. As a result of this experience I had difficulty speaking. Thus I made many mistakes with choice of words. I was having lunch one afternoon with a close friend. She asked me what medications I was taking. Near as I recall, I told her I was taking anticonvulsants Dilantin and Keppra. However, it seems instead of saying Keppra I said Viagra. I was still in recovery and attending speech therapy. I don't think Dr. Kevan VanLandingham wanted me on this medication.

During the first few months of 2002 I realized that more than the seizure focal point was removed from my brain. For the past twenty-five years (as a social service worker, student, and faculty member) I have been very successful at completing several jobs or tasks in a very concentrated time period. I was able to have several client files in operation at the same time. I was able to write lectures and grade homework assignments at the same time. I was able to construct research projects as I did household chores. Against my free will, I believe this multi-task chip was removed from my brain on the day of the surgery on August 15, 2001. It is no longer in my best interest to work on several projects at the same time. I have had to retire that attractive characteristic of my personality. I am best at completing a single task at a time. Perhaps this will change over time as I continue to exercise my brain. But for now, I perform a series of jobs in a row. Only one job at a time. I can no longer perform three or four at a time. Maybe I am closer to my father at this time.

Menopause

I have been seizure-free for over four years. I think my brain has been celebrating this new life. Quite recently I have experienced the early onset of menopause. I am 47 and I am beginning "hot flashes." I think my brain is a bit confused—she thinks she is only a kid and now going through menopause. I think that brain is asking the rest of the body to leave her alone for awhile.

POSITIVE SIDE OF SEIZURES

I think it is time to realize the "positive" side of experiencing seizures. I have been able to describe my weaknesses and accomplishments. I figure as difficult as this time period was, the tortured optimist in me realizes there was a positive side effect of these seizures. I do cheer these at this time.

Never "Wet" Pants

It is quite common for those seizing to lose control of the bladder. I have experiencing at least four grand mal seizures and a few thousand partial seizures over the years. I am quite proud to announce that I *never* lost control of my bladder. I have seen several neurologists in my life and each has asked if I "wet" my pants while seizing. I was always excited to say "no, of course not." Each neurologist told me this was not a guarantee—I could lose control in the future. I had many reasons for deciding to undergo brain surgery. One of those reasons was to ensure that I never lost control of my bladder while seizing. I wanted to maintain this major accomplishment. Of all the times I was embarrassed while seizing I could ensure that I never lost control of my bladder. I'm sure I will have to face that again in the future while aging. My mother tells me I was the easiest to toilet train in my family—I guess I had a strength. I would never lose control during a seizure.

Celebrate Dysfunctional Family

As a Child of an Alcoholic (COA) I learned to follow directions and "orders" from my parents to minimize arguments and disciplinary actions. My family traveled throughout the United States by car during the 1960's and early to mid 1970's. One of the first lessons I learned was to time my bladder on my father's clock. My father was the principle driver from one coast of the country to another. As my father needed, we stopped for food, restrooms, and leg stretches. As a result of these experiences I learned to "hold" as long as necessary. As a result of this experience I was able to attend school all day in junior high school through high school without needing a restroom. This was great as this was the time when smoking started in high school restrooms. I was able to drive from central to northern Illinois without ever stopping to use a restroom.

I have experienced four grand mal seizures and hundreds of complex partial seizures. I never lost control of my bladder. I always thought experiences as a child of an alcoholic offered advantages and expertise. I acquired an additional expertise: I never lost control of my bladder during hundreds of seizures because of experience I received in my family.

THOSE WHO HELPED ME LEARN TO LAUGH

I have always loved laughing. I know endorphins (natural body morphine to cope with pain and sadness) are inspired by laughing. During the past few years I have learned to laugh at myself. Close friends have helped enormously over the years. At school I seek laughter. Thanks for laughing with me and at me. I'm glad I found you all—I stayed above water.

Chapter Eight

Epileptic Zoo
Late Fall 2001

Between ages of 10–20 I declared who I was (1970's)
Between ages of 20–40 I declared what I could do (1980–2000)
Age of 40+ I declared what I could change (2000+)

In November of 2001 I realized that my main focus in life had been coping with seizures. I experienced frightening seizures from 1979 to 2001. Every morning I would wake asking myself "will I have a seizure today? And if I do, how severe will it be?" I can't remember the exact day, but finally one morning in November 2001 my first question in the morning was "what will I experience today?" Finally, the Sociologist jumped out of the shadows—encouraging the epileptic to let go of the "leash." Once again it is time to revisit the past—to seek implications or relationships of events and their connections with the present (Berg 2001). It is time to revisit my four separate "selves" and celebrate the enrichment of their common bonds. Epileptic, meet Child of an Alcoholic—while you're at it, meet Sociologist and Social Services Worker.

The Twelfth Step of Recovery for Adult Children of Alcoholics
(www.geocities.com/howitworks2001/)
    Having experienced the power of growing toward wholeness, we find our bodies, minds and spirits awakened to a new sense of physical and emotional relief which leaves us open to a new awareness of spirituality.

I created the term "epileptic zoo" to describe my life experiences and professions. "Zoo" refers to an artificially reduced habitat, each species fenced off from others. Tilly (1981) adopted this term to describe college or university environments. According to Tilly (1981), professors divide their subject matter and styles of thought into diplomatic, economic, and intellectual divisions. Watching theorists at work is similar to strolling through a zoo: each intellectual species is confined to an artificially reduced habitat, fenced off from predators and prey. Boundaries are real and significant, similar to a zoo (Tilly 1981). Following Tilly (1981) I believe I lived in a self-constructed "epileptic zoo" for over forty years. What I will attempt to do first is describe each species in my zoo. Then I will attempt to describe the creation of my natural habitat. Since 1986 I have experienced three stages of growth toward developing a natural environment. The current stage began during recovery in late 2001—all personal species interact naturally.

Stage One—Creation of the Zoo: Compartmentalization

There were four "species" deposited in the "zoo." It is time to meet each species.

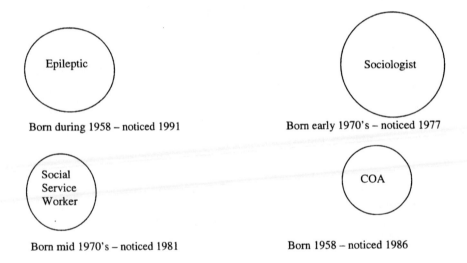

Epileptic
Born during 1958 – noticed 1991

Sociologist
Born early 1970's – noticed 1977

Social Service Worker
Born mid 1970's – noticed 1981

COA
Born 1958 – noticed 1986

Epileptic

The epileptic was born in 1958 but not noticed until 1991. I experienced my first grand mal seizure when seven months old. According to my mother, this seizure was diagnosed as a "convulsion" due to high fever. I experience a few complex partial seizures while in third grade. I didn't know how to describe this experience. I remember coming home from school for lunch one day. All of a sudden I felt my heart beat faster and I began to sweat. I felt nausea and told my mother I felt I had an upset stomach. She told me to stay home from school for the afternoon and go to bed. Ten minutes later I was fine. I was no longer nauseous and felt quite comfortable. I was confused as to why I had to stay home from school that afternoon. I began feeling a few complex partial seizures while in high school—short, rare, and unpredictable. I was never able to describe these events and they were quite rare—until 1980. These events, as described earlier, became frequent and intense in the early 1980's. However, they were not adequately diagnosed and thus lived separately from the other "selves." Eventually, in 1991, the epileptic was noticed: I was formally diagnosed with epilepsy.

The epileptic, during this time, did not interact with the Sociologist, Social Service Worker, or Child of an Alcoholic until 2001. I experienced seizures consistently for the next ten years. However, during this time, the epileptic lived in an artificially reduced habitat. The epileptic was visited each time she experienced a seizure. When the seizure was over, I moved from that "cage" to another. I visited the epileptic many times—only for seconds or minutes. I always convinced myself that each seizure was the last. The epileptic, at this time, did not realize that the Sociologist, Social Service worker and child of an alcoholic helped accept and cope with the condition.

Sociologist

I believe the Sociologist was born in the early 1970's. My family lived in one of northwest suburbs of Chicago. This was an all-white racial suburb. My grandmother lived in downtown Chicago. I clearly remember driving through a variety of neighborhoods before reaching my grandmother's apartment. I was confused why Blacks and Hispanics seemed to live in relatively poor neighborhoods and whites seemed to live in middle or upper middle class neighborhoods. I constantly questioned adult family members of this racial bias. On a regular basis my parents tried to convince me that this was the way neighborhoods were supposed to be constructed. I never bought this argument. It was at this time my mind pondered inequality. I met and saw children/spouses seeming to experience abuse. I saw individuals without appropriate medical, legal, or political intervention based on gender, class, or race. Finally, in 1977, I noticed the Sociologist. I chose Sociology as a major for my Bachelor's Degree. For the next twenty-five years I would continue to question human rights. I began research in the areas of cultural disadvantage, equal medical treatment, political and legal representation, and bureaucratic manipulation. During this period I was not able to connect my beliefs of unfair medical treatment and legal/political representation to my experiences as an epileptic or child of an alcoholic. I could not practice my sociological beliefs as a social service worker.

Social Service Worker

I believe the Social Service Worker in me was born in the mid 1970's. I was sensitive to survivors of social problems. I began pondering social services. Programs should be offered to the disadvantaged. Those experiencing personal problems should be offered support and treatment. During this period I was not able to connect the Social Service Worker in me to my personal background as a child of an alcoholic. I accepted an internship at an alcohol addictions center in Charleston, IL. I loved this internship and was hired as a Counselor aid after I completed my hours. I did not realize that the Sociologist in me questioned bureaucracy of social service agencies.

Child of an Alcoholic (COA)

The Child of an Alcoholic inside of me was born in 1958 but not noticed until 1986. I began working for a mental health center in 1985 as a Substance Abuse Prevention Specialist in Monticello, IL. However, I could not connect the COA in me to my attraction to the field of Social Services. I was working in the field of Addictions and did not connect this to my inability to "cure" my father of alcoholism. Children growing up in an alcoholic household serve to manage the stresses and, as adults, are locked in self-defeating behavior patterns. For example, I had difficulty following projects through from beginning to end, judged myself without mercy, had difficulty having fun, guessed at what normal was, and had difficulty with intimate relationships. I tended to fear change and thus found myself locked into a course of action without consideration of alternatives. I tolerated my life. I dated alcoholics and did not connect this to my experience working with alcoholics. I did not connect the COA to the Sociologist in me questioning healthy families. I never connected the denial of seizures to my family history. I knew my father was an alcoholic but I had never connected his condition to me.

Each Species Visited Separately

Each species was visited separately. While experiencing a seizure I was only an epileptic. While contemplating social problems I was only a Sociologist. While considering social resolutions for the disadvantaged I was only a Social Service Worker. While struggling with my past as the daughter in a dysfunctional family I was only a child of an alcoholic. Each species lived separately for close to twenty years—never sharing resources or common bonds.

Stage Two—1986: First Interaction:
Enter Sharon Wegscheider-Cruse

During the fall of 1986 I attended an addictions conference in Chattanooga, TN. It was during this conference that the child of an alcoholic interacted for the first time with the social service worker inside me.

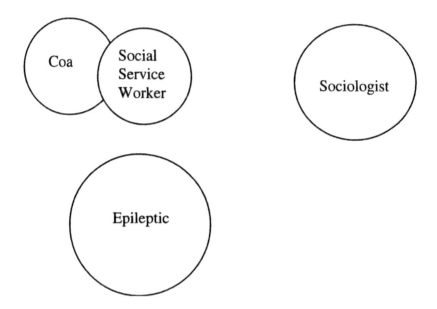

Child of an Alcoholic (COA) Meets Social Service Worker

Sharon Wegscheider-Cruse was the keynote speaker at the Addictions meeting in Tennessee. Sharon described her experience as a Social Service Worker and her history as a child of an alcoholic. It was at this time that the social service worker in me met the child of an alcoholic. As a result of her personal experiences and professional history, Wegscheider-Cruse identified the characteristics of "children of alcoholics." During her keynote lecture, Sharon described the twenty characteristics. For the first time in my life I identified myself as a "child of an alcoholic." This week-long conference was a revelation for me. I realized I was interested in the field of addictions as a result of my experience as a child of an alcoholic. I was not able to encourage my father to stop drinking so seemed interested in "rescuing" other alcoholics from drinking behavior. Finally, I was able to introduce the Social Service Worker to the Child of an Alcoholic inside my soul. This was a significant beginning to my recovery.

Sociologist

The Sociologist inside my soul continued to live separately. I completed my Master of Arts (MA) degree in Sociology in 1986 while working for a social service agency. The Sociology part of my self did not connect with the Social Service Worker. I continued to ponder social problems in our society. I questioned financial decisions made by government and large-scale corporations. I was quite convinced that employees and citizens were manipulated and abused by government and corporations. As a result of continuous manipulation many people may seek counseling at a social service agency. I was not able to formally connect these two ideas. I studied Sociology to understand government and corporate manipulation. I would then begin working with those suffering from social pressures. The Sociologist did not connect with the Social Service Worker.

Epileptic

I continued to experience "feelings" during this time period. I did not know these were complex partial seizures. During the 1980's I began experiencing more frequent and intense "feelings." Each time I experienced a seizure I questioned and endured the experience. However, I continued to believe these were just a "personality quirk." After my negative experiences in 1981 I never told others of these "feelings." I continued to convince myself that each was the last. While experiencing a seizure my other "selves" were not considered. As a child of an alcoholic I received (and internalized) the message "don't talk, don't trust, and don't feel" (Wegscheider-Cruse 1989). I didn't (at that time) realize that the epileptic accepted "don't talk, trust, or feel" and thus never divulged the seizures to others.

In-depth Visits

For the first time in my life I began to connect parts of my sense of "self." As a result of my education and training I was able to connect the Child of an Alcoholic with the Social Service Worker. I was quite aware of the Sociologist aspect of my personality and constantly challenged the decisions made by large-scale organizations which could lead to individual social problems. Thus I began to see the connection between growing numbers of clients in social service agencies with broad institutional philosophy. The broad institutions are education, medicine, government, legal, family, and religion.

Stage Three—1991: Conceptualizing Natural Environment: Enter Gideon Sjoberg

Finally, in 1991 I began to conceptualize a natural environment. I met my future dissertation director Gideon Sjoberg. During the spring of 1991 I was a member of his class on Historical/Comparative Research Models. After several personal discussions I began to note the interaction of my experiences as a Sociologist, Social Service Worker, and Child of an Alcoholic.

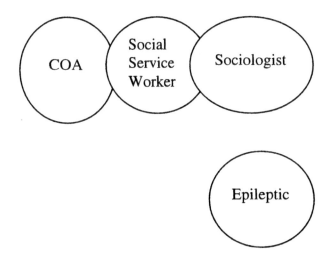

Child of an Alcoholic (COA) Knows Social Service Worker

As mentioned earlier, the child of an alcoholic part of my personality and history connected to the Social Service Worker inside me in 1986. For five years I continued to review my past experiences inside a family surrounded by a history of alcoholism. I continued to follow the twelve-step recovery program. I knew I would not "recover" but always be "recovering." By 1991 I was well aware that my desire to continue in the field of social services was directly related to my experiences in a dysfunctional family. More importantly, I continued to focus on self-growth. As a result, I was ready in 1991 to introduce the Social Service Worker to the Sociologist.

Social Service Worker Meets Sociologist

Per Gideon Sjoberg, I introduced the social service worker to the Sociologist. It was time to connect the spirits of these two. It was Sjoberg's inspiration to search for a dissertation idea which could revise the social service worker and add Sociology. Prior to entering the University of Texas for a Ph.D. in Sociology I had worked for a for-profit social service agency in south Texas. The policy of this facility was to only accept patients carrying private health care insurance covering inpatient care. My job was to construct an acceptable diagnosis to those with insurance and refer those without insurance to alternative settings. I quit this job after 1½ years and entered my doctoral program. Late 1991, the Texas Senate began a three year investigation of for-profit psychiatric hospitals. Through the guidance of Sjoberg, this investigation was the subject of my dissertation. Finally, I was able to connect the Sociologist to the Social Service Worker. The Sociologist questioned for-profit motives of hospitals serving the medically vulnerable. Following the patterns of Sjoberg, I argued that a set of for-profit private psychiatric hospitals "triaged" potential patients. This concept argues that bureaucratic decision makers find it inefficient to treat or work with certain groups and sacrifice their needs is order that others (more beneficial to the organization) can receive services. Private psychiatric hospitals were able to manipulate mentally impaired patients for purposes of profit, thereby leading to exploitation. These hospitals created a supply of patients capable of covering the cost of private care, while at the same time turning away deinstitutionalized patients with genuine treatment needs who had no insurance benefits

The Social Service Worker in my soul had experience in these hospitals and knew what questions to ask, what problems to evaluate, and where to find adequate data. This research connected the Sociologist and Social Service worker brilliantly. Independently, each field was not strong enough for my ideas. Through Sjoberg, I found an intersection of the two fields.

I did not realize this at the time, but the Child of an Alcoholic was dragged into this intersection. I knew I had a history of difficulty following projects through from beginning to end. I also heard rumors that Sjoberg's graduate candidates had difficulty graduating. Sjoberg personally admitted his difficulty closing research or signing dissertations. He was never "satisfied" and thus never completed projects. I refused to be added to this list. Thus, I owned my own history and stepped into my "workaholic" mode and finished the research project on time.

Epileptic

I had dealt with seizures for twenty-five years. I was formally diagnosed an epileptic in the summer of 1991. Although I continued to see neurologists on a consistent basis and follow all medical advice (prescription medications, little alcohol intake, rest) I continued to seize on a regular basis. Eventually I was taking three different medications, experienced severe side effects from each medication, and still experienced 30—90 seizures per month. I accepted this condition. I did not see the connection between my "tolerance" of epilepsy with my experience as a child of an alcoholic. For many years I did not "fight back" or seek medical alternatives. As a child of an alcoholic I feared social change in my own life. I feared that change could make conditions seem worse. Thus, I accepted my epileptic condition for many years. I continued to stay on drugs and experience too many seizures too long. The epileptic continued to exist separately from other aspects of my life. During this time I did not see the interaction between my fear of alternative medical intervention with other experiences in my life.

Noticing the Natural Environment

Following the patterns of Gideon Sjoberg, I began to notice the "natural environment." I was not quite ready to live in this environment but I began to accept this premise as a life-long chore. I was aware that I was a child of an alcoholic, an epileptic, a Sociologist, and a Social Service Worker. These four species contributed to my sense of "self." I was developing my soul based on the years of experience in each of these areas.

Stage Four—2001: Living in a Natural Environment

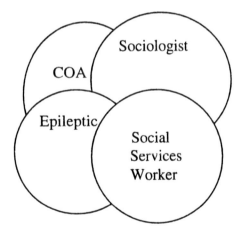

Holism

I am learning to live in a natural environment. Holism versus reductionism is a long-standing debate in the field of social sciences. The concept of holism argues that the whole is greater than the sum of the parts (Sjoberg, Williams, Vaughan, and Sjoberg 1991). Characteristics or actions of a "whole" can not be accounted for by an analysis of individual parts. A "whole" possesses qualities in addition to the sum of the parts. Thus, groups have characteristics or behaviors that individuals do not (Polkinghorn 1983). If one takes the view that the whole is merely the sum of its parts, then rigorous standardization is feasible. But if the whole is conceived as greater than the sum of its parts, then the researcher is obliged to piece together the parts theoretically in order to construct the whole (Sjoberg, Williams, Vaughan, and Sjoberg 1991). Following this pattern, I argue that my natural environment was created by the interaction of my four selves. I can not understand my soul by only looking at the sum parts of each self. It has been the interaction of all four selves that created the whole.

Combining All Four Selves

Without comprehension, I began to combine my four "selves" in the fall of 2001. For the first eight weeks after neurosurgery I was in rehabilitation. Finally, I began to notice the common bonds of all my experiences and accomplishments. I had been experiencing seizures for forty years and for the first time I was able to recognize the positive aspects of this condition. I learned to cope with a physical disability and not allow the condition to stop me from accomplishing goals. I realized I always pressed myself to do my "best" regardless of physical limitations.

I began to realize that it was my experiences as a child of an alcoholic that helped me cope with seizures. I coped for years with my positions in a dysfunctional family. I think the child of an alcoholic helped the epileptic cope with dysfunction. I used this skill to accept my seizures and endure. I learned to love a father with alcoholism. I think this helped me to learn to love myself with seizures.

I chose Sociology as a major my second year of college. I now realize the epileptic and child of an alcoholic tried to understand discrimination and prejudice regarding those with disabilities.

I accepted my first job as a Social Service Worker in 1981. I have worked in a variety of fields offering services to substance abusers, the disabled, and those experiencing social problems. I now see the connection of all of my capabilities. I loved offering support to others because of my own experience as an epileptic and child of an alcoholic. I pursued my Ph.D. in Sociology to continue to study discrimination and prejudice of a variety of groups. My key areas of interest were Research Methods and Large Scale Organizations (particularly Medical Services). The epileptic and child of an alcoholic wanted to study and challenge unfair social trends. Sociology was never enough. The epileptic and child of an alcoholic continued to stay involved with Social Service Organizations. At this time I plan to join a local Rotary Club.

The most common cause of epilepsy treatment failure is noncompliance. Compliance is a multidimensional variable characterized by type of behavior, extent of compliance, and degree of intention. As many as 50% of all patients with epilepsy are noncompliant to a degree that interferes with optimal treatment. Proper management of epilepsy requires physicians to identify noncompliant patients, determine the causes and extent of the problem, and devise and monitor an appropriate intervention strategy. Extent of compliance must be viewed as a continuum of behavior which ranges from the rare patient who takes every prescribed dose precisely as directed, to the consistently noncompliant patient. Most patients fall somewhere between these extremes (Leppik 2000). I was the unique patient—I was the rare patient who took every prescribed dose precisely as directed. I recorded all blood levels, every seizure I experienced, and the length and intensity of all seizures. When it was discussed if I was a surgery candidate, the medical team was quite convinced I was compliant. I think I learned compliance as a child of an alcoholic. I learned to comply with a dysfunctional family. I worked with a variety of populations as a social service worker teaching my clients to comply with standards of care. As a sociologist I research large corporation noncompliance with standards. It was time for me to comply with epilepsy standards to maintain as much control over my seizures as possible.

Living with a seizure condition is difficult. My seizure frequency and intensity increased over the years and I learned tolerance. I coped with discrimination. I dealt with continued embarrassment as seizure frequency and intensity increased. I kept moving forward. I adjusted as a child of an alcoholic—I guess I was ready to adjust as an epileptic experiencing 30 to 90 seizures every month for at least ten years. According to my neurosurgeon (Dr. Michael Haglund), most epileptics have not achieved college degrees or maintained full-time jobs. I learned as a child of an alcoholic to endure.

At this time I wish to acknowledge the positive aspects of living as a "tortured optimist." Following the concept of Gideon Sjoberg (1989) I believe I have always had a positive view of my life in the long run. "Tortured" tended to arrive with respect to the present: my conception of justice and fairness with respect to the way in which organizational power is wielded fails. Brutality of human beings toward one another continues. However, I continued to live as an optimist. I believe this drive pushed me to search for the "best" aspects of all four parts of my self. I continued working the twelve-step recovery program for children of alcoholics. I learned to drop the "don't talk, don't trust, don't feel" model and asked for alternatives. I never stopped trying. I wish to press a message for epileptics and/or children of alcoholics. We can accomplish all we wish. We can turn our "disability" or "dysfunction" into positive and productive functions. Never give up.

Enriched Environment

Current research in zoos has inspired changes in such artificial settings. "Enriched" environments inspire animals to perform more natural behavior and as such improves motivational indices of well-being (Swaisgood, White, and Zhou 2001). Such environments seem to provide a more holistic approach to the enrichment of animals in an artificial zoo (Mellen and MacPhee 2001). "Enriched" environments provide three-dimensional space increasing behavioral repertoires, spacing patterns, and activity budget. As such, a zoo providing a structure or frame which resembles the "wild" significantly increases motivation and "natural" behavior (Ochiai-Ohira and Matsuzawa 2001). Hence, an enriched three-dimensional environment can "naturalize" animals.

I believe I created a natural environment for my four-dimensional personality. A strong argument within the field of Sociology (and other fields) is Holism versus Reductionism. I haven't totally accepted this until now. I survived as a COA, epileptic, Sociologist, and Social Services Worker as a reductionist. Part of recovery was to note the difference between Holism and Reductionism. Finally, after twenty-five years I have created my holistic sense of self.

I was born as a child of an alcoholic. Surviving an alcoholic household led to diligence and tolerance of limitations and deficiencies. Surviving an alcoholic household encouraged me to study Sociology and work as a Social Service Worker. Studying Sociology and working in Social Services encouraged me to accept my epileptic condition and understand deficits as a child of an alcoholic. Survival of epilepsy encouraged me to study Sociology and offer services to the disabled. I learned how to accept and enjoy the components of my life. I can now celebrate the enrichment of common bonds.

Grappling with the Ghost of Sjoberg[1]

Sjoberg's imprint on me was significant. For fifteen years I had been a Sociologist and Social Service worker constantly striving for common bonds. Finally, during the spring of 1991, Sjoberg (my dissertation director) introduced the Social Service worker to the Sociologist. I linked the common bonds of these two fields utilizing the Sjobergian theory of social triage. Although I have rarely met or spoken directly with Sjoberg since graduation, I continue daily discussions reformatting the theory of social triage and considering new research. The theory of social triage argues that bureaucratic decision makers find it inefficient to treat or work with certain groups and therefore sacrifice their needs in order that others (more beneficial to the organization) can receive services. State hospitals discharged large numbers of chronic mentally ill patients to save tax dollars. Private psychiatric facilities denied treatment to the chronic mentally ill to increase profits. The treatment needs of the chronic mentally ill were sacrificed for organizational objectives leading to social triage. Jails and prisons were the only places to take the chronic mentally ill. Research has been strong in the areas of deinstitutionalization, private psychiatric care, and the penal system. However, there has been little research on the connection of these three fields. My current research attempts to expand the theory of social triage to explain a connection between the deinstitutionalization of state hospitals and the increase in the prison population. Thus on a fairly regular basis I find myself arguing with a non-present Sjoberg.

CELEBRATING DUAL DIAGNOSIS AND BACKGROUND EVENTS THAT SHAPED MY HISTORY

Once again I look to Charles Tilly as a mentor. Tilly's (1981) argument was that several social science disciplines have long operated far from history. Tilly's point is that the discipline of sociology grew out of history. Many sociologists did begin to reach for history in the 1970's. Sociological authors noted that when something happened seriously affected how it happened. History began to matter. Time and history moved into practical research agenda. This shift is important. It is enlarging the place of historically grounded theories.

Research has indicated that those with co-occurring "disorders" tend to have significant difficulty recovering from either condition. Thus, those with more than one diagnosis tend to relapse from either condition, have difficulty receiving support, managing funds, securing employment, and acquiring education. Thus, a high percentage of this population tends to become homeless or involved in the criminal justice system (Vocational and Rehabilitation Research Institute; Dual Diagnosis Recovery Network).

In a strange way, I believe my dual diagnosis (epileptic, child of an alcoholic) contributed significantly to my success. I was able to survive and develop the integrated self.

Integrated Self

I used to be Karen Glumm, the epileptic who happened to have a doctoral degree in Sociology. Following Tilly (1981) I argue that it is time for the epileptic to meet the sociologist. In fact, I think the epileptic and sociologist should meet the child of an alcoholic and social service worker. Let's meet them all, for I fully note that when and why something happened grew out of all four of those parts of my life and in turn effected all four.

I believe I have had an enriched life. Experiences as a child of an alcoholic taught me the varying stages of acceptance, love and accept imperfect self and others, and endure dysfunction. As a child of an alcoholic I learned tolerance. I learned to follow orders from parents to minimize disputes. As a family we took an enormous amount of trips around the country by car during the 1960's and 1970's. I learned quite young that we would stop along the highway when my father needed food, restrooms, or to stretch his legs. Thus, I learned to follow his "bladder clock." I was able, throughout the years, to avoid public restrooms (malls, schools, road travel) for up to 12 hours. As a result of this "teachable" moment in my family, I had a tough enough bladder that I never loss control during a seizure.

Education as a Sociologist helped me understand stages of development and inequality in our society. Experience as a Social Service Worker prepared me for personal limitations and alternative treatment. I learned endurance. I continued to exercise my brain through writing, traveling, lecturing, and reading. I have been able to maintain a memory through these exercises.

I am quite proud of my integrated sense of self. Indeed the whole is greater than the sum of the parts.

Recovery Community and Recovery Movement

The "recovery movement" is an organized effort to remove barriers to recovery for those still suffering from problems and to improve the quality of life of those recovering from disability problems (White 2000). The recovery movement offers a challenging invitation: "If you have found recovery, consider giving the community your story as an instrument of hope and healing" (White 2000). It is now time for me to join the fight to expand those resources for those who are still suffering. Public self-disclosure of one's story is just one of a broad spectrum of gifts recovering people can offer to this movement (White 2000). I am an epileptic and a child of an alcoholic. I am not "cured." Relapse is always a possibility—I might seize again. However, I am in recovery and I continue working the twelve steps. It is time to offer services/support to those experiencing epilepsy or those close to epileptics. I plan to encourage epileptics to use a twelve-step recovery program similar to Children of Alcoholics. I will continue an effort to remove barriers and to improve the quality of life of those recovering from addictions or disability burdens. This book is the first of my next 1,000 steps in continued recovery. I would never ask for twenty-five years without seizures. During this time I learned to cope. I learned how to accept who I was, accept limitations, and develop into a new person. My seizure history has its benefits—I can now celebrate the past twenty-five years. I wouldn't trade those seizures for the world.

NOTES

1. Ghost is a former organizational member whose emotional significance was so great, or whose exit was so painful, that remaining members continue to operate as if the person was still in the organization (White 1997).

Summary

"Youth is wasted on Young People"

Mark Twain (Quotations Gallery)

The view on top of this mountain is fantastic—breathtaking. It was worth the climb. I can see, smell, hear, and feel everything.

I have learned to celebrate my strengths and weaknesses. In fact the correlation between these helped me tolerate and survive a seizure disorder. I was born as a child of an alcoholic (COA). Twenty years ago I accepted this label and recognized that I fit all twenty characteristics. Surviving an alcoholic household led to diligence and tolerance of limitations and deficiencies. I obtained a BA, MA, and Ph.D. in Sociology and worked for ten years as a Social Service Worker.

My main thesis is that my twelve-step recovery as a child of an alcoholic taught me to cope with seizures and accept deficiencies. I learned as a COA to tolerate dysfunction and keep family "secrets." I refused to reveal my seizures with friends, attempted to cope with the condition, and eventually pursued treatment and correction. Through Spirituality I acknowledged and accepted my conditions. I endured. I learned to turn dysfunction into function; disability into ability. Furthermore, I have learned the benefits of two diagnoses. I experienced 30–90 seizures per month for the past twenty years but as a recovering COA I never gave up hope for the future. I celebrate the benefits of COA recovery and invite fellow epileptics into a similar 12 step recovery program. I am an epileptic—I will never be cured. I am in recovery.

So, did my life as a child of an alcoholic encourage me to learn Sociology and work as a Social Service Worker? Did surviving an alcoholic household encourage me to keep a journal full of memories and accept my epileptic condition? Did studying Sociology and working in Social Services teach me to understand and accept deficits as a child of an alcoholic and encourage me to utilize tolerance? Did being a Sociologist and working as a Social Service Worker teach me to accept and treat epilepsy? Did survival of epilepsy encourage me to study Sociology and offer services to Disabilities? Did survival of epilepsy encourage me to tolerate a dysfunctional family? I guess this does not matter. It seems I accepted and enjoyed the components of my life. I am Karen Glumm, an epileptic and child of an alcoholic with a Ph.D. in Sociology who worked as a counselor/case manager in a variety of Social Service Agencies. I never let my brain stop working: I continued studying, thinking, writing, traveling, lecturing, and reading. Although seizures continued to increase in intensity I never let my brain die. I continued to play "mind games": exercising my brain. I kept a journal full of ideas and memories.

The optimist inside encouraged me to keep pushing, fighting, hoping, and expecting the best. I endured. I am still seizure-free—that for which I hoped. That optimist is no longer tortured.

It is time to look forward to the future—for the first time in my life I am excited about "tomorrow." Perhaps I feel like "Rip Van Wrinkle"—I was asleep for twenty years. I am now awake trying to make up for lost time. There is a little kid inside of me. Sometimes I am a five year old—low attention span; sometimes eight years old—somewhat mature and enjoying reading; and sometimes I am a teenager—learning life. I enjoy playing, listening to music, reading, talking, singing (only by myself), laughing, listening, and just "being" inside my body. Perhaps this is what Mark Twain implied. I'm a kid at the age of 47. Youth, indeed, is wasted on the young.

Epilogue

I have always been weak on directions. I didn't know the difference between North, South, East, or West (in town walking or driving of course). I have always questioned the origin of this weakness. Did I inherit this from my father? Was I having seizures while being taught or receiving directions? Perhaps I was living so deep in a seizure life-style dark-hole that direction did not matter—as long as I found light. However, directions never seemed to help. Until Kevan VanLandingham and Michael Haglund. Finally, I was led out in the fall of 2001. Direction no longer matters. Light seems to appear in every direction. I am no longer lost.

When I was a child, I learned that our "mind" would never quite remember the feeling of pain. This confused me. However, I learned quite young that this was true. I have experienced physical pain over the years and never remember the true feeling. It seems this type of experience can relate to my seizures. I, for the first time in my life, can not precisely remember the emotional and physical feelings of a complex partial seizure. I have tried but I can not totally conceptualize the experience. So, I drink a toast to my "memory," and to the future of those experiencing seizures. It seems this is an ideal time in medicine for the epileptic patient. Keep fighting, keep trying, keep living—hope is there. Perhaps it is the "tortured optimist" that brought me this far. I'm still walking.

Appendix One

Annual Partial Seizure Report and Accomplishments

First grand mal (generalized) seizure 6/22/91, Early a.m. (in bed asleep)
Second grand mal seizure 7/13/91, 6:00 a.m.—pattern: Dilantin major drug

ACADEMIC YEAR	SEIZURES	ACCOMPLISHMENTS
8/1/91–7/31/92	217 tiny/med/bad 4.6% bad	passed comps, full-time student, counselor at CFS, began dissertation
	added Tegretol	Ph.D. candidacy, TA in Stats and lab
8/1/92– 7/31/93	251 small/med/bad 10% bad	began dissertation, TA in Stats, Data collection, counselor at CFS
8/1/93–7/31/94	353 small/med/bad 10.5% bad	TA Stats, defended dissertation, job search completed, first article written, received Ph.D.
8/1/94–7/31/95	378 small/med/bad 9% bad	9 new classes, Presented at ASA and SSS, Faculty Committee work
8/1/95–7/31/96	368 small/med/bad 14.7% bad	9 classes, Faculty Committees, new research, article published, SSS presentation
8/1/96–7/31/97	389 small/med/bad 11% bad	9 classes, Faculty Committees, ASA and SSS presentation, Committee to develop MHA, Developed/taught MHA class

(continued)

(*continued*)

ACADEMIC YEAR	SEIZURES	ACCOMPLISHMENTS

8/1/97–7/31/98	323 med/bad
	12% bad car
	  accident
	1/23/98
	Grand Mal
	4/14/98 added
	Depakote
		ASA and SSS presentation,
		New research, classes, Committees
		  Graduate class

8/1/98–7/31/99	211 med/bad 16% bad	9 classes, Committees, graduate class SSA presentation
8/1/99–7/31/00	281 med/bad 9/23/99 grand mal 23% bad	9 classes, Committees, SSA presentation, faculty committees,
8/1/00–7/31/01	197 18% bad 8/8 added Keppra	9 classes, Committees, Presented at SSA, Began research on prisons

Spring and Summer 2001—Testing; Surgery on August 14; 8/27/01 and on no seizures

8/1/01–7/31/02	Surgery
	  speech therapy
	  learn to drive,
	  walk
		1 article published,
		1 article accepted for publication,
		3 classes, research on prisons,
		  began book on epilepsy

Appendix Two

Personal Seizure Description

Type	Description
All	Feel on a plain; rise quickly up a mountain; reach a peak; once peak is reached I knew the seizure would taper: decline
Small/Short	Lasts 5–15 seconds; little altered consciousness; no post ictil; possible déjà vu; feel uncomfortable; nervous; can lecture, write, drive, think, remember clearly; immediate recovery
Medium	Lasts 15–30 seconds; post ictil range 0–10 minutes; possible déjà vu, altered consciousness; difficult to lecture, communicate and write during seizure and post ictil; very nervous; uncomfortable; fear; usually stop activity and resume after post ictil; memory may be effected
Bad	Lasts 30+ seconds; post ictil 10 minutes to 4 hours; average recovery is 60 minutes; possible déjà vu; can not communicate (i.e. difficulty speaking and understanding language); must stop activity; extreme fear; very nervous; quite uncomfortable; altered memory; possible headache; try to "swallow" during seizure (swallow seizure?); grasp tightly what is in hands

Glossary

Attention Deficit   a disorder in individuals who have difficulty maintaining an attention span because of their limited ability to concentrate and who exhibit impulsive actions. Provided by On-line Medical Dictionary (Department of Medical Oncology, University of Newcastle upon Tyne, 1997–2002, cancerweb.ncl.ac.uk/cgi-bin/omd).

Aura   A warning that the seizure is about to begin. A sense of "de ja vu," nausea and confusion begin (Epilepsy Foundation).

Child of an Alcoholic   An adult or child who has grown up in an alcoholic family. Children growing up in an alcoholic household often fall into patterns of behavior that, as children, serve to manage the stresses and, as adults, keep the children locked in self-defeating behavior patterns. Adult children are particularly at risk; they learned unhealthy coping behavior at an early age from the dysfunctional family systems in which they were raised. Provided by Sharon Wegscheider-Cruse in *Another Chance: Hope and Health for the Alcoholic Family* (Palo Alto: Science and Behavior Books, Inc., 1989).

Complex Partial   Impairment or loss of consciousness; loss or alteration of consciousness; individual is able to move about in a relatively normal manner but is, at the same time, suddenly lacking understanding; possible amnesia; partially receptive of directions from others; may last a few seconds but usually 1 to 3 minutes; Patients usually experience a period of confusion after the seizure, lasting a few minutes; most patients cannot recall any of the events that occurred during the seizure. Provided by Ilo E. Leppik, MD, in *Patient with Epilepsy* (Newtown: Handbooks in Healthcare, 2000, 5th edition).

Déjà vu

I've seen this before. Provided by Ilo E. Leppik, MD, in *Patient with Epilepsy* (Newtown: Handbooks in Healthcare, 2000, 5th edition).

Depakote

Anticonvulsant medication used to control seizures. Side effects include nausea, indigestion, drowsiness, and hair loss (Eckerd Rx Advisor).

Dilantin

Anticonvulsant medication used to control seizures. Side effects include nausea, vomiting, dizziness, drowsiness, join pain, skin rash, and hair growth (Eckerd Rx Advisor).

Endorphins

Hormone pain relief and euphoria—protein molecules (i.e. peptides) chemically related to opiates, morphine, and heroin that are produced primarily in the pituitary gland and brain. Provided by Christina Gianoulakis, "Alcohol-seeking behavior: the roles of the hypothalamic-pituitary-adrenal axis and the endogenous opioid system" in *Alcohol Health & Research World*, Summer 1998 v22 i3 p202.

Epilepsy

Epilepsy is a neurological condition that makes people susceptible to seizures. A seizure is a change in sensation, awareness, or behavior brought about by a brief electrical disturbance in the brain. Seizures vary from a momentary disruption of the senses, to short periods of unconsciousness or staring spells, to convulsions. Some people have just one type of seizure. Others have more than one type (Epilepsy Foundation).

"Feeling" My personal description of a seizure. Old memories; difficulty speaking or understanding speech; sweating, feelings of fear, confusion, and discomfort.

Ghost (Organizational) A former organizational member whose emotional significance was so great, or whose exit was so painful, that remaining members continue to operate as if the person was still in the organization (White 1997).

Grand Mal Seizure Generally begin without warning. Patient cries out as trunk muscles force expiration of air. Patient suddenly falls to floor from a loss of muscle control. Body experiences contractions. Seizure accompanied by marked increase in heart rate and blood pressure. The seizures last one to two minutes. Incontinence may occur. Full consciousness might not return for 10 to 15 minutes, confusion and fatigue may persist for hours or day. Provided by Leppik in *Patient with Epilepsy* (Newtown: Handbooks in Healthcare, 2000, 5th edition).

"Hard Drive" Brain

Insight Self-understanding as to the motives and reasons behind one's own actions or those of another's. Provided by Department of Medical Oncology of University of Newcastle upon Tyne in *On-line Medical Dictionary* (1997–2002, cancerweb.ncl.ac.uk/cgi-bin/omd).

Keppra Anticonvulsant medication to control seizures. Side effects include weakness, drowsiness, dizziness, loss of coordination, and difficulty walking.

Midlife Crisis A period of emotional turmoil in middle age.

Characterized especially by a strong desire for change. Provided by Merriam Webster's Collegiate Dictionary (www.m-w.com/cgibin/dictionary).

Postictal   Post seizure confusion, recovery; minutes up to days

Privileged vulnerable   Possess a set of resources that are not always
                                   available to other vulnerable groups. This group
                                   may be acutely and temporarily impaired (physical
                                   complications, suicidal, depressed, or other trouble
                                   managing their lives) and thus is vulnerable.
                                   However, this group possesses a set of personal
                                   and social resources (friends, family, physicians,
                                   attorneys) that aid them in their attempts to fight
                                   back against exploitation. This group is fairly
                                   sophisticated and thus possesses knowledge of
                                   hospital and court bureaucracies (Glumm 1994).

Recovery   Patterns of full or partial remission, continuum of
                                   outcomes from its inception. Recovery is the
                                   process of bringing problems into a state of stable
                                   remission. Provided by Bill White in *Toward a
                                   New Recovery Movement: Historical Reflections
                                   on Recovery, Treatment, and Advocacy* (Prepared
                                   for the Center For Substance Abuse Treatment
                                   April 3–5, 2000, Alexandria, Virginia).

Ritual   Any psychomotor activity sustained by an
                                   individual to relieve anxiety or forestall its
                                   development. (Department of Medical Oncology,
                                   University of Newcastle upon Tyne, 1997–2002,
                                   cancerweb.ncl.ac.uk/cgi-bin/omd).

Skeleton in the Closet: Unpleasant secrets, old scandals. Provided by
                                   Wayne Magnuson in *English Idioms Sayings and
                                   Slang* (Prairie House Books 1995-2002, 3rd
                                   version, home.t-online.de/home/toni.goeller/
                                   idiom_wm/).

Social Service Worker   Enhances the lives of individuals with functional
                                   limitations and their families by initiating,
                                   implementing, and promoting quality services
                                   (Coles County Association for Retarded Citizens).

Sociologist

Sociologist conducts studies of society. Sociology grasps a historical time period. *When* something happened will have a strong effect on *how* it happened (Tilly 1981).

Spirituality

Ability to find peace and happiness in an imperfect world and to believe that, even though our own personality is imperfect and the world is imperfect, both we and the world are acceptable. (Wegscheider-Cruse 1989).

Tegretol

Anticonvulsant medication to control seizures. Side effects include nausea, vomiting, dizziness, blurred or double vision, fatigue, and disturbances of coordination (Eckerd Rx Advisor).

Tortured Optimist

Positive view about humanity's prospects over the long run. Sociology can, in its distinctive way, help attain a more humane world. "Tortured" arrives with respect to research of the present: the optimistic conception of justice and fairness with respect to the way in which organizational power is wielded fails. Brutality of human beings toward one another continues (Sjoberg 1989).

Turf

Get rid of, is the essence of the delivery of medical care, the concept of the "revolving door." Provided by Samuel Shem, M.D. in *The House of God* (New York: Dell Publishing, 1988, 3rd edition).

References

Alcoholics Anonymous. (1981). *12 Steps of Recovery.* www.alcoholics-anonymous
.org

Berg, Bruce L. (2001). *Qualitative Research Methods for the Social Sciences.* Boston:
Allyn and Bacon.

Berger, Peter L. (1976). *Pyramids of Sacrifice.* Garden City, NY: Anchor.

CCAR Industries. www.ccarindustries.org

Epilepsy Foundation. Online website. EpilepsyFoundation.org

Gamson, William A. (1992). *Talking Politics.* New York, NY: Cambridge University
Press.

Geocities.com. (2001). *12 Steps of Recovery for Adult Children of Alcoholics.* Geoc-
ities.com/howitworks2001/

Gianoulakis, Christina. (1998). Alcohol-seeking Behavior: the Roles of the Hypothalamic-Pituitary-Adrenal Axis and the Endogenous Opioid System. *Alcohol
Health & Research World,* 22, 202-12,

Glumm, Karen. (1994). *The Social Consequences of Bureaucracy.* Ann Arbor, MI:
UMI.

Goffman, Erving. (1961). *Asylums.* Garden City, NY: Doubleday.

Kubler-Ross, Elisabeth. (1997) [1969]. *On Death and Dying.* New York, NY: Simon
& Schuster.

Leppik, Ilo E. M.D. (2000). *Contemporary Diagnosis and Management of the Patient
with Epilepsy.* Newtown, PA: Handbooks in Health Care.

Lyng, Stephen. (1988). Holism and Reductionism within Applied Behavioral Science:
The Problem of Clinical Medicine. *Journal of Applied Behavioral Science,* 24,
101–117.

Mellen, Jill, and Marty MacPhee. (2001). Philosophy of Environmental Enrichment:
Past, Present, and Future. *Zoo-Biology,* 20:3, 211-226.

Merriam-Webster Inc. (2003). *Merriam Webster's College Dictionary.* Springfield,
MA: Merriam-Webster.

Miller, Mary E. (2002). Seizing Her Life. *News and Observer*, April 21, 1D, 4D, 5D.

Ochiai-Ohira, Tomomi, and Tetsuro Matsuzawa. (2001). Introduction of Two Wooden Climbing Frames as Environmental Enrichment for Captive Chimpanxees and its Assessment. *Japanese Journal of Animal Psychology*, 51:1, 1–9.

Polkinghorne, Donald. (1983). *Methodology for the Human Science*. Albany: State University of New York Press.

Quotations Gallery (2006). Faculty. Quinnipiac.edu/libraries/tballard/quotes.htm

Shem, Samuel. (1978). *The House of God*. New York, NY: Dell.

Sjoberg, Gideon. (1989). Notes on the Life of a Tortured Optimist. *Journal of Applied Behavioral Science*, 25, 475-485.

Sjoberg, Gideon, Norma Williams, Ted R. Vaughan, and Andree F. Sjoberg. (1991). The Case Study Approach in Social Research: Basic Methodological Issues. Pp. 27–79 in Joe R. Feagin, Anthony M. Orum, and Gideon Sjoberg, eds. *A Case for the Case Study*. Chapel Hill, NC: University of North Carolina Press.

Sontag, Susan. (1978). *Illness as Metaphor*. New York, NY: Farrar, Straus and Giroux.

Swaisgood, Ronald R, Angela M. White, and Xiaoping Zhoa. (2001). A Quantitative Assessment of the Efficacy of an Environmental Enrichment Programme for Giant Pandas. *Animal Behaviour*, 61:2, 447-57.

Tilly, Charles. (1981). *As Sociology Meets History*. London: Academic Press.

Wegscheider-Cruse, Sharon. (1989) [1981]. *Another Chance: Hope and Health for the Alcoholic Family*. Palo Alto, CA: Science and Behavior Books, Inc.

White, William L. (2000). *Toward a New Recovery Movement: Historical Reflection on Recovery, Treatment, and Advocacy*. Prepared for the Center for Substance Abuse Treatment April 3-5 in Alexandria Virginia.

White, William L. (1997) [1986]. *The Incestuous Workplace: Stress and Distress in the Organizational Family*. Center City, MN: Hazelden.